Mind Over Meniere's

How I Conquered Meniere's Disease and Learned to Thrive

GLENN SCHWEITZER

Disclaimer:

This book contains the opinions and ideas of its author who is not a doctor or a medical professional. This book is in no way intended as a substitute for the advice of medical professionals. The reader should consult a medical professional before adopting any of the suggestions in this book and in all matters relating to his/her health, particularly with respect to any medications, supplements, and symptoms that may require diagnosis or medical attention.

ISBN-13: 978-1516980925
ISBN-10: 1516980921

For Megan,
Who never lost hope for one second, even when I
was ready to give up. You make me better in every
way. I love you with all my heart.

CONTENTS

CONTENTS

ACKNOWLEDGMENTS

I want to take a moment and thank everyone who helped me shape this book into what it is today. First and foremost, I want to thank my wife-to-be, Megan Jordan, for all of her support, and help with the book. From editing to design, I couldn't have done it without her.

I want to thank my editors and proofreaders, Sharon Taylor-Huppert, and Kari Otto! You both did a wonderful job and made my writing shine. I also want to send a special thanks to everyone who read an early copy of the manuscript. Your feedback and ideas really helped me to write the best book possible.

Lastly, I want to thank you, the readers! When I started the Mind over Meniere's Blog, I didn't really know what to expect. But you all accepted me with open arms, and I watched as an amazing community was born before my eyes. Every day I am humbled by your comments, stories, feedback, and messages. I get so much from you all. Thank you from the bottom of my heart.

FORWARD

Over 69 million Americans suffer from a vestibular disorder. That's a lot!

And yet, most people don't even know what "vestibular" means.

Whenever I share the mission of the Vestibular Disorders Association with someone I've just met, their eyes glaze over at the word "vestibular." So I quickly finish my explanation with, "We inform, support and advocate for people with inner ear balance disorders," and they say, "Oh! I have a friend/family member, etc. who had vertigo."

They get it because I've used terms they understand, and because vestibular disorders are more prevalent than you might think – everyone can relate when it's put in the right context.

But vestibular disorders are not widely recognized and are often misdiagnosed. I can't tell you how many patients I've spoken to who relay the same horrific story of how they went from doctor to doctor, over a period of months or years, and were told that their symptoms were all in their head, or that there is no effective treatment for their condition.

Our vestibular system gives us the sense of where we are in space. When this system is damaged due to illness or injury we lose our ability to balance. Vestibular disorders often cause hearing loss, tinnitus (constant ringing in the ears), nausea, fatigue, and cognitive problems. They can also result in social isolation, inability to work, and loss of independence. But worst of all, because they are invisible to others, many people don't understand the debilitating impact a vestibular disorder can have on the life of a patient and their family.

That's where this book comes in. Glenn has lived the vestibular nightmare. He understands the challenges vestibular patients face every day, and he has learned to live a full and productive life with a chronic vestibular disorder.

In *Mind Over Meniere's*, Glenn shares his personal story. He confesses his deepest fears, then tells you how he overcame them.

Glenn is enthusiastic and entrepreneurial. He stumbles, then he finds a way to deal with the challenges he has to face as a result of Meniere's disease. Glenn offers many helpful tips and tools for the vestibular patient from his own personal experience. And he offers hope.

This book is an excellent resource for vestibular patients who are struggling to accept their limitations, and who are looking for concrete solutions to help them move forward with their life.

If you struggle with dizziness or imbalance, you are

not alone.

While there are many different types of vestibular disorders, and each patient has a slightly different experience, there are also many common threads – grief, frustration, loneliness, fatigue, and brain fog, to mention a few. Glenn offers many different coping strategies. Take what fits and apply it to your life. Even if you are already on the road to recovery, there is always room for improvement.

Wishing you balance,

Cynthia Ryan, MBA
Executive Director
Vestibular Disorders Association (VEDA)

INTRODUCTION

My equilibrium failed me. I sat in horror as the stable world I had always taken for granted deserted me, suddenly and without explanation.

Am I sick? Did I eat something bad? All I had eaten for hours was a bag of Chex Mix.

My mind reeled. Off in the distance, I heard my professor say, "Okay, now open your text book to page 151..." I had no idea what we were learning. It was something about manipulating a computer database. I couldn't bring her words into focus.

As the world began to spin around me, vision doubling, I thought, "How am I going to get home?" There was still 30 minutes left in the class.

I started sweating through my shirt. I had been getting dizzy for months with no rhyme or reason. Not like this though. Never like this.

I was in my senior year at Florida Atlantic University in Boca Raton, Florida, as a business/IT major. I had everything going for me and my future looked bright, but now this.

"What's wrong with me?" The thought desperately echoed through my mind for the rest of the class. No answers came. The answers wouldn't come until much later.

After I got home, the ceiling finally stopped moving. I lay in bed as my mind drifted back to the ten-minute trip home I had taken hundreds of times before. I should never have driven home. Driving drunk would have been safer.

As the room settled back into the stable reality I knew and loved, my 24-year-old self shrugged the whole thing off. I was still invincible back then. I would have to suffer for a while before any answers would come. And a bit more after that, as well.

That was just the beginning. A terrifying start to what has now become a four-year journey. I didn't know it then, but I was suffering from Meniere's disease. A chronic condition of the inner ear that causes tinnitus (loud ringing), feelings of intense ear pressure, hearing loss, and "attacks" of violent vertigo. There are many theories, but modern medicine has yet to find a cause or discover a cure.

What started as an imposing life sentence has slowly evolved into a journey of self-discovery. In the months and years that followed, I took back my health piece by piece. Today I find myself healthier in mind, body, and spirit; healthier than I've been in a long time.

If you have just been diagnosed with Meniere's disease or are currently suffering, I want you to grasp one thing right now: there is so much hope. Meniere's disease will not define you. It cannot and will not ever be bigger than your dreams. I wish someone had told me this sooner. It may be hard to see it right now, but you can regain much of what you have seemingly lost and have the opportunity build a life of purpose and meaning more substantial than you ever dreamed possible.

I will show you the way through the confusion you undoubtedly feel. You will be able to face your Meniere's disease without fear or hesitation. I will help teach you to take back control of your lifestyle and health with simple and effective techniques. With a little bit of effort, you will come out the other side stronger, happier, and more confident. You will thrive once again.

This book is divided into three sections. The first section will gently guide you to an understanding of Meniere's disease. Early on, I suffered needlessly. I will steer you through the chaos to avoid the crippling anxiety and depression that many Meniere's patients tragically face. Through the combination of knowledge, proper mindset, and finding the right doctor, you will replace your despair with a sense of confidence and hope. It will pave the road for acceptance, your first true step towards health.

The second section offers a system of lifestyle management techniques that will bring you back toward a baseline level of health. Before you can thrive, you need to get your symptoms to a more manageable level. Facing a challenge like that alone can be a frustrating cycle of trial and error, but it doesn't have to be. It's also frightening to face the prospect of having to make massive changes to your lifestyle (giving up coffee was the hardest for me). The good news is that many of the lifestyle changes you face are only temporary, a necessary evil to allow yourself to accurately discover your body's new limitations. As you start to rediscover your health and begin to thrive, you will find that your limitations will constantly change and may decrease over time.

I will also teach you how to build routines that automate aspects of both your mental and physical health to allow you to easily transition into your temporary new lifestyle. Diet, exercise, sleep, and stress reduction all play an important role in treating Meniere's disease and will help manage your symptoms when approached the right way.

The final section will feature a roadmap for you to advance your health further and begin to thrive. You will carefully test what your body can and cannot handle by conducting what I call lifestyle reversal experiments. You will learn how to reach states of optimal experience and peak performance, called flow states, which will reveal potential that you never dreamed possible. I will cover cognitive boosting supplements, called Nootropics, as well as techniques that will help you cut through the brain fog and increase your memory and focus. You will also learn various strategies for personal growth and techniques for ongoing lifestyle management as they relate to Meniere's disease. And finally, I will show you how to find purpose, passion, and clarity in your life. It's not as difficult as you might think.

In fact, if you are anything like me, you may have overestimated the challenges in front of you. It will take hard work, discipline, and courage, of course. Yet far too often, we have a tendency to exaggerate the level of difficulty involved when facing large obstacles.

You are capable of incredible things; nothing is impossible. As you take your first steps, I want you to know you are not alone. There is so much hope. You will thrive again.

Part 1:

Understanding

MY PERSONAL STORY

It was mindless suffering. Without a label to define my situation, I was lost and most certainly in denial. My earliest memory of dizziness stretches back four months prior to my eventual diagnosis. My girlfriend Megan and I were on a whirlwind tour of Los Angeles, California. We came to LA with two days to explore the city and visit friends before driving down to a wedding in San Diego.

We wanted to see it all, driving around in our bright yellow late '90s Dodge Neon rental car. After a quick breakfast of iced coffee and pastries on the Santa Monica pier, we set off to see as much of the sprawling city as we could. Ten minutes away, our first stop was Venice Beach.

As we pushed through the crowds of people and street vendors along the Venice Beach boardwalk, I noticed something was off. Dizziness wasn't the right word. I felt fuzzy, like I was walking through a dense haze. In hindsight, this was my first run in with the phenomenon of brain fog, the ever present clouding of consciousness that dominated my journey early on. It was shortly after this that the dizziness first showed up.

I had started to drive us away from Venice Beach but pulled over after a few short blocks. I was filled with

9

anxiety, my stomach in knots. I was too dizzy to focus on the road. Megan would have to drive us for the rest of the vacation. From that point until well after my diagnosis, the dizziness would wax and wane but never go away.

In the months that followed our trip, a clear pattern began to emerge. Clear at least to Megan. I was still stubbornly set in denial. I was getting dizzy so often, but every time it passed, I would dismiss it, convinced that whatever had caused it either went away or would reveal itself in time.

I have also suffered from anxiety for most of my life. Deep down, I know that this is what drove my denial. To go to the doctor meant the possibility of there actually being something wrong. The irony is that getting help sooner could have significantly reduced my suffering. But at the time, denial was just so much easier. Things would have to deteriorate for a few more months before I would resign to the inevitable. My suffering began to escalate, slowly but surely.

Several weeks later, after a delicious steak dinner, Megan and I had gone out for some coffee and dessert when suddenly, my stomach lurched. As panic took hold, I ran to the bathroom. Ten harrowing minutes later, I shivered on the floor in the bathroom of the local coffee shop. Tears streaming down my face, the waves of nausea were starting to pass, but the bathroom was still spinning. I could barely stand up. I fumbled for my phone and texted Megan to come to the bathroom immediately, that something was wrong.

As soon as she opened the door, her look of horror said it all. I had been violently sick, not even making it to the toilet before the succumbing to the nausea. It had to be food poisoning. I was dizzy and nauseous and felt completely drained. I don't know why, but at that moment, all I could feel was shame. I didn't want her to see me like this, but I needed her. She helped me clean myself up and drove me home. I never ate at that restaurant again. In reality, it was just a very sodium-heavy meal that triggered my symptoms, but I was convinced otherwise at the time. I warned my friends and family not to eat there. I still hadn't made the connection.

I kept telling myself I was going to be fine. Every day, there was dizziness and a new denial. My ears felt like they were filled with fluid, but I didn't have a cold. "Lower your voice!" became Megan's anthem. I didn't know I was yelling. I would soon learn that my hearing was affected. Megan had been pressuring me to see a doctor for weeks now. I guess I wasn't ready to let the problem become real. But everything was about to change. What happened next was undeniable.

It only took an instant to break me. It was 8pm on January 31st, 2012. Nothing was particularly remarkable about the first twenty hours of that day. I finished classes at 7pm and grabbed dinner on the way to

Megan's apartment. It was around 74 degrees, a beautiful South Florida winter day. We mindlessly watched old sitcom reruns as we ate.

As I finished my bacon cheeseburger and fries, I stood up to throw away the trash. But as I walked back to the couch, warning bells were literally sounding off in my head. My ears were ringing, louder than I ever imagined possible. A sharp pressure ramped up in my right ear. My stomach somersaulted as equilibrium swiftly dropped away. I fell onto the couch and couldn't get up. I couldn't move as intense nausea washed over me. Once again, panic took hold as the room spun faster and faster. Megan sat and tried to comfort me, gently rubbing my hair. "It's going to be ok. We're going to get you help." The shadowy shape of a problem that had followed me for months finally became solid as intense vertigo took over.

The world stopped spinning forty-five traumatic minutes later. My armor of denial destroyed, piled up in the corner. I collapsed on the bed; I had never known exhaustion so complete. My life force drained of all reserves. I promised Megan I would make a doctor's appointment the next day and let the last bit of my waking consciousness fade to black.

The next day, I woke up in a state of confusion. I felt like I had been in a car accident. A thick haze blanketed my mind as memories of the previous night's ordeal trickled back into my awareness. I had suffered my first full blown vertigo attack. Everything else up to that point had paled in comparison. Luckily, Megan had the day off and was still home to take care of me. I called my parents to let them know what had happened. They knew about some of the dizziness I had been dealing with for the past several weeks and were scared, but happy I was going to get help. I hung up and pulled up my health insurance provider's website on Megan's laptop. I brought up a list of local ear, nose, and throat (ENT) doctors and called the one closest to Megan's apartment. I was able to make an appointment for later that afternoon. But it was a mistake, and one I've made before. I chose a doctor out of convenience and not reputation. I was in for a rude awakening. A doctor's personality and mindset can make or break you. I was about to be broken again.

The doctor's office was in a medical complex several blocks away from Megan's apartment. My mind still felt like scrambled eggs, and I was scared. As I waited to see the doctor, I tried to put the pieces together. Nothing made sense. I had never experienced anything like this in my entire life. As I went over the previous day's events in my mind one final time, they called me back into the exam room.

The doctor was an older gentleman. His expression was sterile, emotionless. He asked me what was wrong. I decided to start with last night's vertigo and work backward. He listened intently, but I couldn't read his face or guess what he might be thinking. I explained the feeling of pressure in my ears, the ringing, and the ever present, but fluctuating, dizziness. When I finished, he was still writing down notes in my file. After a moment, he set down his pen and nodded sternly.

"You have Meniere's disease. It affects the inner ear and causes all of the symptoms you've just described. The exact cause is unknown, but it results in the dizziness, mental fatigue, vertigo, and all of the symptoms you are experiencing. There is, unfortunately, no cure. Every time you have an attack as you had last night, your hearing will be permanently damaged, though only slightly. One attack won't change much but over time will result in a total loss of hearing. I'm going to write you a prescription for a diuretic and a corticosteroid. These will help the symptoms. You have to eat a low sodium diet, no caffeine, nicotine, or alcohol and try to avoid stress."

I was swallowed whole by an anxious abyss; so much for avoiding stress. My mind raced away from me in fragments; incurable, going deaf, change everything, helpless. It was so much worse than I ever could have imagined, and it was delivered in the cold way you would imagine only a robot capable of. It gets worse.

When I don't understand something, I tend to ask a million questions. It's been this way as far back as I can remember. So when facing something as confusing and traumatic as an incurable, debilitating, medical diagnosis, I did what I've always done. I asked a million questions. I just wanted to understand, needed to understand. The doctor didn't see it this way. He didn't see the terrified, trembling young man in front of him whose world had just been turned upside down. He saw only a questioning of his intelligence and let it be known.

The doctor said, "You don't believe me? Are you questioning my expertise? You have Meniere's disease. You have to make these changes. It's the only way. Are you the doctor now?" I couldn't believe what I was hearing. I tried to explain, "You just told me I have an incurable disease. I just want to understand. You said I had to change everything but didn't explain why. I'm not questioning your expertise. I'm just trying to understand!" He didn't get it. I left that day beaten, scared, and hopeless. I started into a slow spiral of depression. The following week was one of the lowest points of my entire life. Worse yet, it was entirely and completely unnecessary. At the time though, I had no hope. I was trapped in the fixed mindset of my bitter and emotionless doctor.

The experience rocked my worldview to its foundation. I didn't know what to do with myself. I didn't change anything at first in a final last ditch effort of denial. The prospect of a lifetime of continuous suffering was still too big to grasp. For the next week, I continued to drink coffee, eat normally, and avoided the medication I was prescribed. Needless to say, nothing changed except my state of mind. It was now painfully obvious that my doctor was right. My depression deepened.

It was a hard pill for my family to swallow, as well. Most people have never heard of Meniere's disease, let alone understand it. They tried their best to be supportive, but what they wanted most was for me to get a second opinion. I was indifferent, having already resigned to my seemingly inevitable fate. My grandfather was able to get a referral to a specialist at the University of Miami, about an hour south of where I lived. I was miraculously able to get an appointment ten days out. In the meantime, however, I had started to test the suggestions of my first doctor. I lowered my sodium intake and switched to decaf coffee. I also started the regimen of prednisone (a pharmaceutical steroid) and Diazide (a diuretic). Unfortunately, I stopped sleeping as a result.

The prednisone made it hard to fall asleep, and the diuretics woke me every hour to go to the bathroom. The lack of sleep was compounding my depression and anxiety. Despite this setback, the feeling of fullness in my ears was starting to dissipate. The dizziness was becoming more subtle, as well. It was promising. I still felt hopeless but began to realize I had some measure of control. Looking back, I see now that this was my first turning point, a running start that opened my mind enough to receive what happened next.

I became very strict with my sodium intake, keeping it between 1500mg and 2000mg per day. I stopped taking the diuretics and did my best to get at least 8 hours of sleep. I slowly started exercising, little by little, and sought alternative treatments like acupuncture. I was also overweight at the time and relatively unhealthy in other aspects of my life. At the very least, I realized I could improve the rest of my health to give myself a fighting chance.

I also stopped researching my symptoms on the internet. After my doctor's appointment, I read everything I could possibly find about Meniere's disease, but I was filling my head with horrible reports of the worst cases of suffering. People who successfully overcome their major health problems are not generally the ones who write about it on the internet. Researching symptoms and negative reports filled my mind with terrible expectations and caused negative, self-fulfilling prophesies. As a general rule of thumb, if what you are reading doesn't leave you with a sense of optimism, avoid it. It may be doing you more harm than good.

As the days passed, my symptoms slowly improved. Little by little, I started to allow myself to have hope. Everything came to a head when, at last, I finally saw the specialist.

I drove down to the University of Miami hospital,

feeling grateful that I wasn't too dizzy to drive. I was nervous but hopeful. As a well-known specialist of hearing and balance disorders, the doctor had treated a large number of Meniere's disease cases. More importantly, he came highly recommended.

I waited for about forty-five minutes, filling out paperwork in the large crowded waiting room of the Otolaryngology wing of the hospital. A friendly nurse eventually led me to a small exam room and took my vitals. A student in residency at the hospital came in next. After explaining everything that had happened over the last several months, he agreed it sounded like Meniere's disease and said he was happy to hear I had been proactive about my health. Finally, some thirty minutes later, the doctor arrived and his demeanor quickly put me at ease. In stark contrast to my first doctor, he was kind and compassionate. He confirmed it was most likely Meniere's disease but wanted to have an MRI, another audiogram, and several other tests done to be sure. He was patient and answered all of my questions. He knew I was scared and painted an optimistic picture. He told me that though lifestyle changes are needed to get the symptoms under control, there was no need to think anything was permanent. He explained how the disease tends to change over time and can lessen as your body adapts. He shared success stories of several of his other patients. He told me all the changes I had made so far were the right ones and to keep up the good work. He reassured me that if I was able to get my symptoms under control and stop having attacks, my hearing would most likely never be lost and that everything would be ok. Without question, he saved my life.

He filled me with the hope I desperately needed. I now felt potential where before there was only fear. I saw the world through a new lens, a new mindset. He gave me my power back. It brings tears to my eyes thinking back to this defining moment. It was like a light switch went on in my head. Meniere's disease would never define me. It didn't have the power anymore. It makes me shudder to think of what my life might have looked like had I never met him. Finding the right doctor changed everything for me.

I drove home a new man. For the first time, I saw clearly the obstacle that blocked my way. I knew I faced an uphill battle, but there was a solution, a way forward. My new doctor gave me this gift. With a surging confidence, I saw the bigger picture and, with a smile on my face, I knew I would be ok in the long run. What had first seemed like an impossible challenge, was now an opportunity to learn and grow as a person. As I write this, years later, I see with perfect clarity the amazing direction my life took from that point forward. Given the path I was on, I know I would never have grown to be the man I am today otherwise.

GLENN SCHWEITZER

ACCEPTANCE

It has been an interesting several years since my diagnosis. Looking back, it's clear that acceptance is the first step on the path to health. Unfortunately, our capacity for denial can seem limitless, especially when our health is at stake. When facing such a seemingly massive challenge, your mind will try to reject whatever happens to be causing you stress. This response is a natural defense mechanism and exists for a good reason. Denial is there to protect you and give you the time you need to adjust to a painful or stressful issue. But if you never process what you're going through, there is a point where denial becomes another obstacle that must be addressed. Fortunately, there are several ways to make this easier.

When facing your diagnosis, you may have the same initial reaction that I had, that what your doctor has told you simply can't be true. If you are anything like me, you will probably try to make a last ditch effort of denial, hoping your symptoms will magically disappear. This is a natural impulse, and one I thoroughly understand. It's okay to feel this way. If you feel the need, like I did, to test your diagnosis, then here is a simple way to do it.

Think of this process as an experiment, with a clear

start and end point. Give yourself no more than a week and don't change anything in your lifestyle. First, grab a blank notepad or journal and jot down today's date as the starting date and one week from now as the end date. Twice a day, once in the morning and once in the evening, write down an honest assessment of your symptoms and how you feel. When the week is over, go back and read all of your entries from start to finish. If your symptoms stay the same or get worse, then it's time to take action. Keep in mind, however, that this whole process is unnecessary, especially if you have already found a doctor you trust.

Finding the right doctor is possibly the single most important thing for you to do early on. It is a powerful force to move you towards acceptance and eventually health. But the wrong doctor can be your undoing. Start by answering a few simple questions about your current doctor:

- How is your doctor's bedside manner? Did he approach your case with compassion and kindness? My first doctor didn't, and it caused me a lot of unnecessary pain. This quality is crucial to your treatment.
- After you saw your doctor, were you left with a feeling of hope or were you filled with hopelessness? The answer speaks to your doctor's mindset and, as a consequence, your

mindset.

- Did your doctor answer all of your questions? It's important to feel that your doctor is on your team. If he isn't supportive in this way, you may be left feeling like you're all alone.
- How did you feel when you left after your appointment? If you felt unsettled or unsure about your doctor in any way, don't hesitate to find a new one.

Finding the right doctor will make every step of your journey easier and sets you up to succeed. First, though, it's helpful to understand some of the basics. Doctors who specialize in treating ear conditions are called ear, nose, and throat physicians, or ENTs for short. This branch of medicine is called Otolaryngology. Many ENTs will have a basic understanding of Meniere's disease and may even have some experience treating patients, though this not their area of expertise.

After completing ENT training, a doctor can choose to become even more specialized. A neurotologist is an ENT physician who specializes in treating inner ear conditions that affect hearing and balance. You have the best chance of finding a great doctor by seeking out neurotologists in your area. They will have the most experience in treating Meniere's disease. You can check if your doctor is a board certified neurotologist through the American Board of Otolaryngology website (Aboto.org/ABOInternet/VerifyPhysicianCertification).

The Vestibular Disorders Association Provider Directory (Vestibular.org/finding-help-support/provider-directory) is another excellent resource, allowing you to search for doctors by location and specialty. Both are good starting points but don't factor in the doctor's personality. Fortunately, you can find this out with a little bit of research.

Over the last several years, doctor rating websites have sprung up all over the internet. But one stands out above the rest: Healthgrades.com. Not only can you search for doctors by location and specialty, but you can find patient satisfaction information, as well. Patients fill out anonymous surveys that cover the entirety of their experience with a doctor, and Healthgrades aggregates the surveys into a single rating score. You can also find information about the doctor's practice, facilities, possible malpractice suits, awards they've won, the conditions they treat, and much more. It's an empowering website. If I had known about Healthgrades sooner, I could have easily found the low rating of the first doctor I saw. It would have saved me considerable pain. A quick search for neurotologists in your area will get you started.

Lastly, when looking for the right doctor, having a referral can be a huge time saver. Even if you don't know anyone else who has Meniere's disease, you have options. The US News and World Report, for instance, has a ranking of the top ENT hospitals in the United States (Health.usnews.com/best-hospitals/rankings/ear-nose-and-throat). You can often get a referral to a great doctor in your area by calling the Otolaryngology department at these hospitals. You also can go back to Healthgrades and seek out highly ranked neurotologists in other locations. Most would be happy to refer you to a local specialist if they know of one. Keep in mind, though, if you live in a remote area, there may not be a specialist nearby. If this is the case, start with the best ENTs in your area, but know that travel might ultimately become necessary to find the right doctor.

I highly recommend getting second or even third opinions, as well. Getting multiple opinions will help you to move towards acceptance, even if you end up staying with the first doctor for treatment. It also increases the odds of finding the doctor that best matches your personality. Even if you liked your first doctor, you might find the second one to be a better fit.

The last piece of the puzzle has to do with mindset. In her bestselling book *Mindset: The New Psychology of Success*, Stanford psychologist Carol Dweck lays out her groundbreaking research on the power of our beliefs and how small changes in understanding can lead to big results. Dweck describes two distinct personality types that ultimately define a person's belief system: the "fixed mindset" and the "growth mindset."

A person with a fixed mindset believes their character, personality, intelligence, creativity, and talent are unchangeable and set at birth. If they are naturally smart or possess talents, they must avoid failure at all costs as a way to maintain their sense of superiority. When faced with failure or setbacks in life, a person with a fixed mindset reacts poorly and tends to blame others to avoid improvement. Whereas a person with a growth mindset believes no traits are fixed; that talent, ability, and personality are goals, achieved through hard work and dedicated effort. A person with a growth mindset views failure and setbacks as opportunities for learning and growth. Obviously, having a doctor with a growth mindset will be hugely beneficial.

The first doctor I saw had a fixed mindset. When I asked him questions, he got angry. Instead of seeing a scared patient who needed hope, he saw a kid who questioned his intelligence. His mindset prevented me from seeing even a glimpse of a future where I might be okay. It's a stark contrast to the second doctor I saw. He exuded hope and optimism. He clearly painted a picture of a future where I could thrive and, as a result, I eventually did. As you search, keep in mind that your doctor's mindset will be contagious. It's important for you to view Meniere's disease as only a setback, an obstacle in your path to be overcome. A doctor with a growth mindset will help you see that. As a result, you will grow and develop as a human being. You will learn to be in touch with your body and mind on a much deeper level.

Hopefully by now you have reached some level of acceptance. You have Meniere's disease. You can't change that, so now what? Now, you focus on everything you can change. The Stoic philosopher Epictetus once said, "Happiness and freedom begin with a clear understanding of one principle. Some things are within your control. And some things are not." You still have control over most aspects of your life. Discovering the right places to focus your energy will give you the best chance of success. First, though, you need to have a basic understanding of Meniere's disease. Only then can we begin to identify the ideal focal points for your attention and efforts.

GLENN SCHWEITZER

UNDERSTANDING MENIERE'S DISEASE WITHOUT FEAR

Trying to understand Meniere's disease can be frustrating. It is an idiopathic disease, meaning its cause is unknown, and there is no consistent definition among experts. It also doesn't help that there are no tests that can conclusively diagnose Meniere's disease. The only way to know you have it is to rule out all other possible causes of your symptoms. As a result, it's challenging to pin down a good definition of Meniere's and a terrible starting point for any new patient trying to educate themselves.

To make things simple, I've distilled a basic description. Meniere's disease is a chronic condition where patients experience one or more of the following symptoms:

- Rotational vertigo, where it feels as if the room is spinning
- A feeling of fullness or pressure in the ears
- Progressive, but fluctuating, loss of hearing
- Hearing sounds and tones when there are none, commonly known as tinnitus

The symptoms tend to occur as individual episodes

that vary in intensity and duration, though symptoms can persist between episodes. During an episode, a patient may also experience nausea, fatigue, difficulty concentrating and recalling words (otherwise known as "brain fog"), or a host of other symptoms. An episode can last anywhere from minutes to hours and typically leaves people feeling completely exhausted when it's over. These episodes, or "attacks" as I referred to them previously, are terrifying, especially when you don't know what's causing them.

Facing a Meniere's disease diagnosis is overwhelming, there is no denying that. As I write this, there is currently no cure or even a clear understanding of what causes it. Each episode of Meniere's disease damages your hearing slightly, and over time, can destroy your hearing entirely. Additionally, you will never get a diagnosis without having symptoms. So if you know you have Meniere's disease, then you already know what it means to suffer. You may be in pain right now.

It's hard to be optimistic when facing such adversity. Understand though, it's not the life sentence it may seem on the surface. By making changes to your lifestyle, you can quickly begin to improve your symptoms and learn to live in harmony with your disease.

You will be able to discover what triggers your symptoms as well as what helps you to feel your best.

With a proactive approach, your hearing will be protected; there is no reason to expect to go deaf if you no longer have vertigo attacks. It will take courage, but it's worth the effort. You will not only get better but learn to thrive as you begin to understand your body and your health at a level you never imagined possible. There is so much hope, but it's easy to forget that.

Once you have a basic understanding of Meniere's disease, it's better to focus on the road to health and finding the right levers to pull to get you there.

But before we dive into lifestyle management, I want to shine a light on what will most likely be a big factor in your recovery: everyone else. Having a strong support network will be essential to your treatment. It can get complicated, though. For starters, most people have never heard of Meniere's disease. By most estimates, Meniere's disease only affects about 0.2% of the population. Odds are, the people closest to you will have never heard of it. And worse, Meniere's disease is invisible; no one will recognize your pain at first glance. People will have a hard time understanding what you are going through. People may also underestimate the severity of your symptoms. This can be incredibly frustrating. Having clear communication with your family, friends, and colleagues is important, especially when you are suffering. You will probably have to explain yourself to others more often than you would like, or should have to for that matter.

Only you will ever truly know how you feel, but those closest to you will have a better idea than most. Helping them understand Meniere's disease and your specific needs will create a strong foundation of support for you to build on. In your most vulnerable moments, when you are feeling hopeless and suffering the most, they will be the ones to catch you and get you back on your feet.

Early on, Megan was my rock. In the weeks after my diagnosis, I was a mess. Megan had watched me suffer for months, and I know she felt powerless to help, but she was always there for me. While I was convinced my life was over, she never gave up hope, even for one second. She gave me the strength I needed in my darkest moments. Having an educated support network, with a growth mindset, will keep you moving in the right direction when you're ready to throw in the towel. They will be there, ready to fill you with hope when you need it most. Take the time to set up even the simplest support network and it will pay dividends; you will never be alone on your road back to health.

As you prepare to fight this battle, remember, there is so much hope. I will show you the way. You will not resign to living in defeat. The way forward is one of action and growth. You are not trapped by your Meniere's disease. Let's begin.

Part 2:
Lifestyle Management

TEMPORARY LIFESTYLE OVERHAUL

Welcome to the first step of your journey. However bad your symptoms might be right now, know that just like everything else in life, it will change eventually. The Greek philosopher Socrates once said, "The secret of change is to focus all of your energy not on fighting the old but on building the new." So in this spirit, the first step is to be proactive and temporarily overhaul your lifestyle.

Make no mistake about it, change is hard, even on a temporary basis. But compared to what most patients are led to believe, that they must immediately make permanent and sweeping changes to their lifestyle, a temporary change is a much easier pill to swallow.

The lifestyle overhaul is designed to help you manage your symptoms in three simple steps:

1. Eliminate the triggers of your symptoms
2. Discover the things that make you feel amazing and add them to your life
3. Implement lifestyle management techniques to improve all other aspects of your mental and physical health

When you have a Meniere's disease episode, whether a full blown vertigo attack or otherwise, it may seem to have happened randomly, but that's not usually the case. Something triggered your symptoms. There are many common triggers for a Meniere's disease episode, but they vary from person to person. Knowing your individual triggers will be an important part of your treatment.

The best approach for treating your Meniere's disease is to eliminate, temporarily, all of the well-known triggers while taking steps to clean up your lifestyle to improve the rest of your health. It's much easier to identify your individual triggers by removing them first and adding them back in later on, rather than the reverse. It will improve your health faster and help you identify the things that benefit you.

Having a solid foundation of health will improve your results. A healthy body can fight off illness much more efficiently than an unhealthy body. If you are physically unhealthy and out of shape, a portion of your immune system's resources will be unavailable, stuck dealing with other issues.

Common Triggers

Before you can ever learn to thrive, you will need to get your symptoms and health back to a more manageable level. Learning to listen to your body is the first step. By paying close attention to how you feel throughout the day and keeping detailed notes, you will discover your triggers and identify your new limitations.

When I was about ten years old, I went in for allergy testing and found that I was mildly allergic to milk. For a while, my parents changed my diet. Over time, though, it seemed to affect me less and less until eventually I forgot about it.

Fast forward about seventeen years, when out of nowhere, I started having strange symptoms that triggered my Meniere's disease. At random, I would get a runny nose and, with it, dizziness and brain fog. It went on for months. I had no idea what was wrong with me until one night, Megan and I were out at the local comedy club. While we waited for the show to start, we ordered an ice cream sundae. We ate our sundae and watched as more people filled the club. But fifteen minutes later, my nose started running and I felt impaired as brain fog settled in. It didn't make any sense. That night as I fell asleep, my mind suddenly made the connection, and it jolted me awake. It came as a rush. It was the ice cream... the milk!

I thought back to the last couple of months, and the pattern was suddenly clear. My milk allergy had come back and was triggering my symptoms. I couldn't believe it had taken me so long to figure it out. But this sort of missed association happens all the time. Most people just aren't very good at making these connections naturally. There is, however, an easy way around this shortcoming. A simple practice, as old as time: writing in a journal.

When we have the right information in front of us, we're very good at finding patterns. Keeping a journal will give you the information you need to quickly identify the triggers of your symptoms. Your journal will serve as a daily record of your symptoms and store specific information on your lifestyle. Being able to reflect back on your day, any time you start having symptoms, will speed up the process of finding your triggers. Very quickly, patterns will emerge that will give you a much better understanding of Meniere's disease and your specific triggers. It will also help to identify the things that make you feel great.

Journaling will play an important role in many different aspects of your treatment. Throughout the book, I will describe various journaling strategies, each with its own benefits. But to make journaling and finding your triggers as easy as possible, I have created a one-page PDF journal tool to help you keep track of your lifestyle and symptoms. Get your free copy at: Mindovermenieres.com/journal.

Now let's explore the most common triggers of Meniere's disease. If you have already seen a doctor, you are probably aware of what seems to be a big trigger for the majority of Meniere's cases: salt, or more specifically, too much sodium in your diet.

There are many theories as to what causes Meniere's disease. Some people believe it has a viral cause, while others believe it could be the result of an autoimmune condition. There is also some preliminary research that suggests that there is a genetic component in a small percentage of cases. But one of the more common theories states that Meniere's disease is caused by an increase in fluid and pressure in the endolymphatic chamber of the inner ear. As the pressure builds, the thin vestibular membrane that surrounds the endolymphatic chamber can rupture, causing the fluid to flow over and mix with the fluid in the neighboring perilymphatic chamber. This unnatural mixture is believed to cause vertigo. And because sodium causes the body to retain fluid, high sodium levels are thought to increase the fluid pressure in the inner ear. Whether this is the actual cause of Meniere's disease or not doesn't matter. What matters is that reducing sodium intake can reduce symptoms for a large majority of patients. It helped me considerably.

Caffeine is another common trigger. Giving up coffee left me heartbroken. Most doctors will tell you to avoid caffeine. What most doctors won't tell you is that you may be fine with caffeine in moderation. But it's important to eliminate it initially during your temporary lifestyle overhaul. Once your symptoms are under control, you may find you can tolerate a cup of coffee or two perfectly well.

Nicotine, another stimulant, is also a big trigger. If you are a smoker, you will need to quit, not just to eliminate nicotine, but to reduce the negative impact of smoking on your overall health. It's incredibly important. I quit smoking using nicotine gum and lozenges. It wasn't easy, but I discovered a few things that helped. When I had a craving for a cigarette, the impulse was to smoke, not to chew a piece of Nicorette gum. The reality, however, was that if I chewed a piece of nicotine gum instead, the craving would go away. The trick was to convince myself to chew the gum first. Every time I had a craving, I would tell myself, "If the gum doesn't help in the next ten minutes, I'll have a smoke." But it always helped, and after about a week, I was able to start weaning off the gum.

Picking a firm quit date is important, too. Set a date, tell your family and friends, and stick to it. Your support group will be able to help keep you accountable and give you extra encouragement when you need it the most. I know how hard it is to quit smoking, but it's necessary. As an experiment, I tried chewing a piece of nicotine gum a few months after my diagnosis and immediately got dizzy. I spit it out before my symptoms got worse.

Alcohol is another common trigger. You may come to find that alcohol doesn't affect your symptoms, but it's important to hold off for a while and not drink any alcohol until your symptoms are better controlled. If you find that alcohol is a trigger for you, there are some interesting natural alternatives that I'll explore in the final section of the book.

Like alcohol, many recreational drugs are also triggers. I don't condone the use of any illegal recreational drugs, yet I know they are a part of our society. During the initial lifestyle overhaul, avoid recreational drugs completely, including marijuana, even though it is now legal in several states.

As I discovered with milk, allergies and food sensitivities are extremely common triggers for a lot of people. You may also find the reverse to be true, as well, that Meniere's disease can cause your allergies and food sensitivities to get worse. Either way, finding the connections between your allergies and your Meniere's disease will be important. Journaling will help you find the patterns, but allergy testing is a good idea. It will save you time and take out the guess work. Strictly avoid anything you know you are allergic to during the lifestyle overhaul. Take an antihistamine like Cetirizine (Zyrtec) during the day if you are allergic to anything that can't be avoided, like pollen or dust. Your doctor may also want to prescribe you something stronger if over-the-counter antihistamines are not enough.

Unfortunately, there are also several common environmental triggers of Meniere's disease that are entirely outside of your control. These can include changes in the barometric pressure, changes in the weather, pollution, bright lights, certain types of inflammation, and the visual sensory overload that can happen in places like shopping malls and grocery stores. If you find that your symptoms are triggered by forces outside of your control, or worse, if you find that your symptoms aren't triggered by anything specific at all, don't give up hope. You can still improve your symptoms by focusing on the triggers you can control, or at the very least by improving the overall level of your health.

The last several triggers I will mention have to do with lifestyle. Stress and sleep deprivation are big triggers for a lot of people. Both play a significant role in your health, as well. Stress comes in all shapes and sizes. Having an argument with your significant other. Working with a manager who breathes down your neck. Having a new child on the way. The list is endless. We can't control most of it either. What we can control is our response to stress. Learning to manage stress will be crucial to your progress. Sleep is just as important. Getting a full night of quality sleep is one of the most powerful tools at your disposal to overcome Meniere's disease. Sleep deprivation, on the other hand, will not only trigger more Meniere's episodes but will also disrupt all other aspects of your health. Sleep will play such an important role in your treatment. I can't emphasize this enough.

Change is never simple. But there is a technique that makes it a lot easier. When trying to develop new habits, it's much less stressful if you have a routine to follow. In the early days of my diagnosis, having a routine made everything so much simpler for me. It was my security blanket. It took away the need to make constant decisions, saving my brain's precious resources.

We have only a fixed amount of energy to make decisions during the day. The more energy we waste making small, insignificant choices, the less we have available to make important ones. This phenomenon is commonly known as Decision Fatigue. Our ability to make good decisions deteriorates as we make decisions throughout the day. In a *New York Times* article titled "Do You Suffer from Decision Fatigue," journalist John Tierney explains: "No matter how rational and high-minded you try to be, you can't make decision after decision without paying a biological price. It's different from ordinary physical fatigue — you're not consciously aware of being tired — but you're low on mental energy. The more choices you make throughout the day, the harder each one becomes for your brain..."

With this in mind, it is better to automate your lifestyle changes by following a routine, rather than making continuous decisions throughout the day.

My routine didn't develop all at once. As I

discovered things that helped my symptoms, it slowly evolved. It started with sleep. I went to bed and woke up at the same time every day. I still do. Next, when I discovered how much exercise seemed to help, I added it to the routine. I went to the gym at the same time every day. I ate my meals and snacks at the same time every day, as well. Whenever I discovered anything that helped reduce my symptoms or increase my well-being, I added it into my routine.

Following a routine will also help you discover your triggers. If you keep everything else in your life constant, then when you make a change, you can clearly see the effect of that change. Developing a fixed routine will help you build the momentum you need to succeed. It will also help you to have better communication with your doctor.

Throughout your treatment, your doctor may prescribe a variety of medications for you. It may be similar to what I received, a diuretic and a corticosteroid such as prednisone, though there are many other medications your doctor may want to try.

Diuretics are prescribed to reduce fluid retention with the hope of improving the fluid balance in your inner ear. Steroids are prescribed to reduce inflammation in the inner ear, again, to improve fluid balance. It's important to take whatever medications your doctor prescribes for you. But it's even more important to communicate with your doctor and let him know how they are affecting you. All drugs, prescription or over-the-counter, have side effects. The diuretics helped reduce my symptoms but completely ruined the quality of my sleep. When I brought it up to my doctor, he decided sleep was more important at this stage and had me stop taking the diuretics. Both your routine and journaling practice will help you to accurately report back to your doctor.

The rest of this section will explore specific lifestyle management techniques in much greater detail. I will bring together concepts of health and lifestyle through the lens of Meniere's disease in a novel way. I will introduce you to a wide variety of effective strategies to help improve your symptoms, the first of which is to optimize your diet.

DIET

"Let food be thy medicine and medicine be thy food." – Hippocrates

Eating great food is one of the most pleasurable aspects of life. Is there anything quite like enjoying a delicious meal with family or good friends?

Food is a powerful force in our lives. It can be an experience, a bridge between cultures, or a way to socialize. It can make us feel nourished or drain us of our energy. At a deeper level, food affects our body and mind in a much more tangible and physical way. Like medicine, food causes changes in our bodies at the chemical level. We don't think of our diet this way very often, but it doesn't make it any less real. Food has the potential to heal us. A poor diet, however, can quietly degrade our health.

If you eat an unhealthy diet, you may not even realize that your health is impaired. It becomes your normal state of existence. But it's actually having a profoundly negative effect on your physical and mental health, whether you notice it or not.

It doesn't help that the quality of the food supply in most developed countries has largely deteriorated over the last several decades. Heavily processed and unhealthy ingredients such as high fructose corn syrup dominate our grocery store shelves. Most produce is grown on massive single-crop commercial farms, drenched with fertilizer and pesticides. Most meat is produced in similar, large-scale factory farms, where the animals are pumped full of antibiotics and fed an unnatural diet of corn. In the US, we are facing an obesity and health epidemic of mind-boggling proportions. The complexity of our food system is enormous and, for a Meniere's sufferer especially, there are several major implications and important things to consider.

Eating a Low Sodium Diet

When starting the lifestyle overhaul, it's important to reduce your sodium intake. A high sodium diet will trigger symptoms for a large percentage of Meniere's cases. Most ENTs will suggest this strategy. Check with your doctor first, but aim to reduce your sodium intake to a daily total of 1200mg to 2000mg. Of course, this is much easier said than done. You have to constantly check your food for sodium content, and it takes time to develop an awareness to the point that you don't have to check everything all the time. It's also important to spread out your sodium consumption over the course of your day. One sodium heavy meal, even if you are within your daily limit, can be enough to trigger your symptoms. Try to spread out the 1200-2000mg you consume as evenly as possible. I learned this the hard way.

My first doctor only instructed me to restrict my sodium intake to 2000mg daily, which I did, but I still had symptoms. Basically, I would eat whatever I wanted within my daily limit. But at some point I realized that one sodium heavy meal was all it took to trigger me. As soon as I started spreading my sodium consumption evenly throughout the day, my symptoms started to improve.

Your first line of defense is the FDA required nutrition label on packaged food products. Understand that there is sodium in just about everything. Get in the habit of checking the labels on everything you purchase at the grocery store. The amount of sodium will vary from brand to brand, so always make sure to compare. Sometimes, you will only have to switch brands to maintain a lower sodium diet.

When you do your grocery shopping, keep in mind that the vast majority of the packaged products are processed foods. Anything that comes in a can, box, or bag, has a long list of ingredients, or is frozen or dehydrated, is most likely a highly processed food product. Aside from being less healthy, most processed food products are very high in sodium and should be avoided.

You have to be especially careful with sauces,

dressings, marinades, dry rubs, and condiments. They are all typically very high in sodium. Also be careful when selecting the following: bread, cheeses, yogurts, soups, canned meats, tuna fish, cold cut deli meats, crackers, cookies, chips, and cereals. If it seems like you have to be wary of just about everything, you're right. But it gets easier to navigate with time.

Premium and gourmet grocery stores, such as Wholefoods and Fresh Market, will have a much wider selection of low sodium options, especially when it comes to snack foods. If you can afford it, doing your grocery shopping at these premium stores is an excellent strategy. In addition to having more low sodium options, they usually have a large selection of local and organic foods, as well. If not, purchase your low sodium products at the premium stores, and do your general food shopping at the local grocery store. Farmers markets are another great option. They're usually cheaper than the premium grocery stores and have a wide variety of fresh produce and meats.

When you sit down to eat, it's important to realize that every single part of the meal has sodium, and often it's the little things that can put you over the top. Let's take a look at how a simple meal breaks down. A slice of bread or dinner roll usually has 100-250mg of sodium. Assuming you used unsalted butter, that's 5-15% of your daily sodium intake before the meal even officially begins. Next, you have a simple garden salad.

Most salad dressings have 200-500mg of sodium per serving. Finally, the main course consists of marinated and grilled chicken breasts. Most marinades have more sodium than the saltiest salad dressings. Very quickly, this one meal can add up to more than 50% of your daily sodium allowance.

This is just one simplified example. Most of the time, your meals will be more varied than this. You may also have sides and a dessert. That diet soda you drank? It has sodium, too. Even if your main course is low in sodium, everything else can add up. You have to factor the entire meal into your calculation. It's hard initially but gets easier as you go.

Snacking is another interesting challenge. Most snack foods at the grocery store are high in sodium. Chances are you'll find "reduced sodium" and "low sodium" snacks, but often this is misleading. You have to check the packaging to be sure. My general rule of thumb for safe snacking is to find snacks that have 80mg of sodium per serving or less. But it's worth it to find snacks that you enjoy that have 20mg or less. The serving size of many snacks is smaller than you think. Most likely the serving size was determined to make some other aspect of the nutrition label more appealing. The 100 calorie sized snacks are a perfect example of this.

If you can find great tasting snacks that have 20mg of sodium or less, you can snack without fear. You won't have to worry about eating more than the serving size or making a significant dent in your daily allowance. At premium grocery stores, you can often find a wide variety of options with 20mg or less. To give you an idea, some of my personal favorites are unsalted potato chips, unsalted trail mix, and banana chips. Following this snacking strategy made a huge difference in my mindset. Eating healthy is important, but knowing which snacks you can safely enjoy is empowering.

Your sense of taste may be an obstacle initially as well, especially if you are used to eating a higher sodium diet. Removing salt from your cooking can make your food seem bland. Interestingly though, research has shown that our taste for salty food is, in fact, an acquired taste. If you are struggling with the low sodium diet, know that the cravings for salt go away over time. Higher sodium foods you used to enjoy will start to taste terrible. You will know immediately if food is too salty for you to be eating. You will also find you have a new appreciation for the foods you enjoy. You will start to notice the flavors of the actual ingredients. I consider myself a foodie. I love to go out and eat amazing food. Eating low sodium may have restricted some of my options, but it has only increased my love and appreciation for a great meal.

To add some flavor to your cooking, you have some interesting options. One great trick I discovered early on was to use a small pinch of the spice called "Old Bay" instead of salt. Growing up in Maryland, I've had Old Bay on food for most of my life. It has a bold, salty, and spicy sort of taste that makes most people think of blue crabs but tastes great on a wide variety of food. It has sodium, but 2/3 less than table salt, and its strong flavor means you can get away with using very little.

Many other spices and ingredients can make up for salt, as well. Salt has an acidic taste, so finding and using other acidic ingredients is an excellent strategy. One perfect example of this is lemon. With either fresh lemons or lemon zest, you can achieve a savory flavor similar to salt. There is also a wide variety of salt-free spice blends. For example, Mrs. Dash Seasonings can be found at most grocery stores in many different flavors. There are also many artisan spice companies that produce gourmet, sodium-free spice blends. A quick Google search for "salt free gourmet seasonings" will give you a good list of choices.

As you experiment with taste in the kitchen, make sure to keep notes of what works well. Some other great ingredients to explore are cumin, rosemary, lemongrass, star anise, thyme, cilantro, coriander, gomasio (made from ground and dry roasted sesame seeds), basil, garlic powder, black pepper, onion powder, cayenne, and tarragon. There are endless flavor combinations to try. Be adventurous.

Keep track of your sodium intake in your journal.

Make sure to write down everything you eat and the total sodium content of the meal. You may not know exactly how much sodium is in every single component of your meal, but you should be able to at least make an educated guess. It doesn't have to be perfect. Remember, you are looking for patterns and trends over time.

Eating Out with a Low Sodium Diet

Going out to eat, whether at a restaurant or dinner party, comes with a whole new set of challenges. But with a little bit of planning, you can still go out and enjoy yourself. Most restaurants will happily accommodate for dietary restrictions. But keep in mind, chefs love to cook with salt and will often use a lot of it. So asking for less salt is a bad strategy. It doesn't mean anything specific. It will probably still be too much. Instead, ask if they can prepare your meal without salt, including the sides. If they can't do it, they will let you know. Usually, it's either because the meat has been pre-seasoned or the sides have been pre-made.

Some restaurants will have fewer options, but if you are going out with friends, don't let that hold you back. I've never been to a restaurant that didn't have at least one low sodium option. I find fish to be a great universal choice. Even if all of the chicken and red meat entrees are pre-seasoned, you'll find most restaurants prepare fish to order and can make it for you without salt. But when in doubt, order a salad with plain or lightly seasoned grilled chicken and have them bring olive oil and balsamic vinegar on the side. When you order your food without salt, make sure to let your waiter know it's important. They are well aware that many people have dietary restrictions and will never be upset with you for making the request. Also, when asked, most servers will be happy to make a recommendation for the best entrees that can be cooked without salt.

I've found that big chain restaurants are the hardest to eat at. There are usually very few low sodium options available. On the flip side, the rise of the "farm to table" restaurant has been a godsend. These restaurants serve delicious, local, fresh, and healthy meals. I have several nearby, and at most of them, virtually nothing is off limits.

The worst choice, however, that you can make in restaurants is fast food. It's best to avoid it entirely. Even the salads can have over 1000mg of sodium once you factor in the dressing and meat. In my experience, little good can come from eating fast food when you have Meniere's disease. The combination of highly processed and unhealthy ingredients, loaded with sodium, is a recipe for disaster. To get better, you need to start eating healthy. There is no room for fast food with this approach.

Eating Low Sodium When You Travel

For me, the hardest challenge with restaurants has always had to do with travel. When you are on vacation, you are probably going to be eating out at restaurants for every meal. The best way I've found to manage this is to use tools like Yelp.com, TripAdvisor.com, and Google.com to research restaurants and menus ahead of time. Once you have picked out the restaurants with the most accommodating menus, you can quickly and easily book reservations with Opentable.com.

Take the time to plan out your meals before your leave for your trip. It will save you a lot of stress and disappointment, and it makes for a much more enjoyable trip. Aside from the initial planning, you'll also have to be disciplined throughout the entire trip. Indulge and enjoy yourself, but make sure to keep your sodium intake in check. Nothing ruins a vacation faster than vertigo.

If you are going to the airport or are going to be out for most of the day, make sure to bring healthy snacks with you. It can be hard to find low sodium snacks on the go.

Eating Low Sodium at Dinner Parties

If you're going to a dinner party, the strategy is a little bit different. If the host doesn't know about your low sodium diet, your best option is to let them know ahead of time. Most people will be happy to cook a small portion separately without salt for you. But if this isn't possible, you still have options. In this situation, I typically eat something before I leave, and bring a small snack with me. During the meal, I'll usually eat a small portion to be polite. If you are eating with family or good friends, ask them to cook the food without salt. They may not do it, but never be afraid to ask. Most people are happy to salt their food at the table before they eat.

Every once in a while you may find yourself in a situation without any good options. A wedding with a buffet, for example. If you can pull a server aside, they may be able to speak to the chef and find out which option has the least sodium. Otherwise, the best you can do is to try to use your sense of taste to figure out the safest choice.

If you overdo it and trigger your symptoms, don't be too hard on yourself. As long as you are extra careful with your sodium intake over the next couple of days, you'll most likely be ok.

Prepared Meal Delivery Service

In the last several years, a new type of food business has popped up throughout the US. The basic concept is simple: get pre-made and properly portioned, healthy, gourmet, and fresh meals delivered to your front door, every couple of days. Not all of these businesses will be able to accommodate a low sodium diet, but if you can find one that does, it can be a lifesaver. It was for me. I had a hard time maintaining the low sodium diet. Finding a meal delivery company that could accommodate me changed everything. It not only gave me a wide selection of delicious food to eat, but I was finally eating healthy. It helped me to get in shape and also relieved me of having to make decisions about my meals every day, freeing me up to focus on other areas of my health.

Expect to pay roughly between $5 and $10 per meal, plus a possible delivery fee. You can find out if there are any companies near you by searching for "healthy meal delivery service around (your address)" and "healthy meal plans around (your address)" on Google.

Healthy Eating

While lowering your sodium intake is your first priority, eating healthy is a close second. It won't have as drastic of an immediate impact on your symptoms, but it will improve your health and make all of your other efforts more effective. You can't change the fact that you have Meniere's disease, but you can change the rest of your health. You have complete control over what you put into your body. By getting in shape and eating a healthy diet, you will give your body the strength it needs to deal with your symptoms. If you are unhealthy, your body will have to spend its precious resources elsewhere.

The problem is that there are thousands of books written on healthy eating with wildly conflicting approaches. Author and psychiatrist M. Scott Peck once said, "We know a great deal more about the causes of physical disease than we do about the causes of physical health." Our bodies are infinitely complex biological systems. There are so many variables involved with physical health that it's impossible to identify a universal set of rules that, when followed, result in a healthy human being. Every individual person has a unique body and brain chemistry. And what works well for one person, may not work for others.

But with the intention of treating Meniere's disease, I will lay out some basic concepts and general principles for eating healthy. First, however, understand that being healthy starts with making a choice; the choice to live a healthy lifestyle. It simplifies your treatment by giving you a clear guideline for making decisions. All you have to do is ask yourself, is this choice I am about to make the healthy choice? Hopefully in time, living a healthy lifestyle will become a core part of you. It most certainly has for me.

One major point of confusion surrounding the food industry seems to be the debate of "organic versus conventional" produce and meats. At the grocery store, you may have noticed how some of the produce is labeled organic, while others are labeled conventional or not labeled at all. So what exactly does it all mean?

According to the USDA, "Organic farms and food processors: preserve natural resources and biodiversity, support animal health and welfare, provide access to the outdoors so that animals can exercise their natural behaviors, only use approved materials, and do not use genetically modified ingredients." Simply put, organic food is grown in a sustainable and natural way, without the use of harmful chemicals. Conventional food, on the other hand, is not produced with these limitations. Most conventional farming is done on massive single crop industrial farms that require heavy use of chemical fertilizer, pesticides, and herbicides.

The use of genetically modified organism (or GMO) crops is another fiercely debated topic within the food industry. GMOs are crops that are genetically engineered to contain specific traits that are not found in nature, but achieve one or more of the following goals: increase the food output per plant, increase drought resistance, create herbicide resistance, or create pesticide producing factors. But at the time of writing this, the long term effects of eating GMO foods are still largely unknown.

I advocate eating organic foods whenever possible. This, however, has less to do with the controversy surrounding GMOs and more to do with conventional farming practices. The fertilizers, pesticides, and potentially toxic herbicides like Glyphosate (Roundup) inevitably end up in the food supply. In my opinion, and from the standpoint of Meniere's disease, the fewer toxins we're exposed to, no matter how insignificant the amount, the better chance we have of fighting our illness. Processing toxins from our body requires resources and immune function. While this may not be noticeable in a healthy adult, for a Meniere's sufferer, it can negatively affect your treatment efforts.

The meat industry faces a similar controversy. The vast majority of meat production in the United States is appalling. Take cows, for instance. Cows are raised in gigantic commercial feedlots known as concentrated animal feeding operations, or CAFOs for short. Thousands and thousands of cows are packed tightly into overcrowded pens for the majority of their lives. In his bestselling book *The Omnivore's Dilemma*, Michael Pollan writes, "There is another cost to raising cattle on CAFOs, one that's even harder to see. These animals have evolved to eat grass. But in a CAFO they are forced to eat corn—at considerable cost to their health, to the health of the land, and ultimately to the health of us, their eaters. What keeps a feedlot animal healthy— or healthy enough—are antibiotics. Most of the antibiotics sold in America today are for animal feed, not for humans. Without these drugs, cattle could not survive. The only reason they need the drugs is because they are being raised on factory farms and fed corn."

The question most people never ask is, "What did my food eat?" You will not get healthy by eating unhealthy animals. The same holds true for produce. Spinach grown in iron-depleted soil will not magically produce iron on its own. Eating poorly raised food over a long period of time will cause a cumulative and negative effect on your health. For someone with Meniere's disease, this should be avoided.

As an alternative, try to find meats that are labeled USDA organic, grass-fed, or pastured (not to be confused with pasteurized). Cows that were raised on a pasture and ate a natural diet of grass will generally be labeled grass-fed at the supermarket. Not only is this the more humane way to raise the animals, but in all likelihood, the animals were far more healthy. The meat will be much leaner, much healthier for you, and in my opinion tastier. The only downside is that organic and grass-fed meats tend to be more expensive. But if you can afford to purchase in bulk directly from a cattle farmer and fill up your freezer, it can often be purchased for much cheaper prices. This holds true for dairy products, as well. Look for grass-fed milk, butter, yogurts, and anything else produced from milk. Chicken and pig farms face the same issues; look for organic, pastured, or free range pigs, chickens, and eggs whenever possible. If you live in Canada or the US, check out Eatwild.com/products/ for a directory of over 1400 pasture-based farms, many of which offer their products in bulk and at a discount.

Another byproduct of the industrialized agricultural system is the use of highly processed ingredients. Corn and soybeans are the most prevalent crops grown in America by far. Both are heavily subsidized by the government and, as a result, we have a huge supply of excess corn and soybeans with prices being driven down. Most of the corn, however, is not the delicious corn on the cob you're used to enjoying at the family barbecue. It is a high yield corn that is rock hard and inedible. The corn is broken down into its chemical constituents and turned into processed food ingredients used by food manufacturers. High fructose corn syrup is one example. Because the cost of corn is so cheap, it's often less expensive to use high fructose corn syrup than sugar in food manufacturing. As a result, more and more highly processed, but less healthy, sugary food products are appearing on grocery store shelves on a regular basis. It's also why companies like Coca-Cola now use high fructose corn syrup in their sodas: to make a greater profit.

The sugar content of your food is another factor you need to pay attention to. Sugary foods can trigger vertigo and other symptoms in some people. But even if it's not a trigger for you, it's still important not to overindulge. I believe that the rising sugar content of our food supply is one of the main reasons for the obesity epidemic in America. When you eat a meal with a lot of sugar, your blood glucose levels spike. The spike is followed by a crash. The crash triggers food cravings, which start the vicious cycle all over again. Make sure to eat a diet that is low in sugar. But at the same time, know that it's ok to indulge in moderation. It's important to enjoy life and treat yourself from time to time. Keep track of your sugar intake in your journal alongside your sodium intake. You might be surprised to find there is a connection between your sugar intake and how you feel, Meniere's symptoms aside.

Putting the quality of our food aside for a moment, portion size is another variable to consider when eating a healthy diet. In America, we have a long tradition of overeating large and relatively unhealthy meals. If you want to be healthy, it's important to eat a more reasonable amount of food.

I don't have any specific rules to offer you, but I do have some general guidelines. If you are left feeling uncomfortably full after every meal, you are eating too big of a portion size. You want to be comfortably satiated, not stuffed to the gills. Eating slowly can help you achieve this goal, though it's something I constantly struggle with. For some reason, I always tend to eat like it's a race. I have to consciously slow myself down or I end up eating too much. I encourage you to take this approach, as well. It takes about ten to twenty minutes for your stomach to signal your brain that you are full. If you eat too fast, you won't even realize you're full, and you will certainly overdo it. Overeating also causes a stress response in the body that can trigger your symptoms. Make a concerted effort to eat moderately sized portions at a nice slow pace.

If you continue to eat a healthy, minimally processed diet, it will pay you dividends throughout your journey. Your symptoms will improve faster and it will make a huge difference in how you feel on a daily basis. You will have more energy, mental clarity, strength, and an overall sense of well-being. It will be the foundation to build on as you learn to thrive. Make healthy eating a goal to continually work towards. You will never be perfect, and that's okay. It's about moving forward, making good decisions, and keeping a healthy mindset.

Journaling and Your Diet

Your journal is your secret weapon against Meniere's

disease. It ties all of your treatment efforts together and gives you a clear picture of your progress. Unfortunately, food can affect how we feel hours, or even days, later. With Meniere's disease, the wrong foods can trigger our symptoms. To avoid this, you need to identify your dietary triggers as soon as possible.

There are several great journaling strategies to help you make the connections quickly. First, it is important to keep a food log in either your journal or with the PDF journal tool I provided. Keep a detailed record of everything you eat, especially for the first few weeks. Write down the sodium and sugar content for everything. Make this part of your daily routine. Every time you eat a meal, take a few minutes to update your food log and make sure to include any snacks you may have had in between meals.

The other piece of information you need to keep track of is how you feel throughout the day. Three times a day, once in the morning, once in the afternoon, and once in the evening, write a detailed description of how you feel in your journal. List any symptoms you are experiencing and how severe they are. If you feel good, make sure to write about that, as well. By discovering what makes you feel great, and adding more of it into your life, you will speed up your journey back to health.

Once you have some data to reflect back on, you will

start to notice patterns. Any time your symptoms get worse, analyze what you ate that day and the day prior. When you see a possible connection, make a note of it. You can quickly test potential dietary triggers by eating the food again, and waiting to see if you have the same reaction. If you do, immediately eliminate it from your diet. You may be able to add it back in later on, but for now, eliminate it. Remember, the goal here is to identify everything that triggers your symptoms and eliminate all of it temporarily. This is crucial. The faster you can eliminate your triggers, the faster you will return to health.

You may also find connections between the foods you eat and the way you feel that have nothing to do with Meniere's disease symptoms. Food affects your body and mind in a very real and physical way. People who don't have Meniere's disease can also get brain fog if they eat a poor diet. Ultimately, the goal is to optimize your physical and mental health as much as possible. Journaling will help you get there.

In addition to managing your diet, you also need to be able to manage your stress. Stress can trigger your symptoms in a big way. While a healthy diet helps to improve your physical well-being, effective stress management will improve your mental well-being. In the next chapter, I will teach you several powerful techniques to reduce your stress and improve your mindset.

STRESS AND MENTAL WELL-BEING

"He is most powerful who has power over himself." – Seneca

As we go about our lives, we all experience stress in one form or another. It's a fundamental part of life. We evolved a stress response for a good reason. When faced with a dangerous situation, we need to be able to react quickly. Humans may be at the top of the food chain today, but it's not because of our physical strength. Throughout history, most predatory animals could quickly overpower us. It's our brain, our capacity to think, that gives us our great advantage. So to deal with environmental threats, humans evolved a stress response, commonly known as the fight or flight response, to quickly prime the body to respond to danger.

In today's modern world, we don't face the same physical threats as our ancestors did. Yet the stress response still exists. In small doses, stress isn't a problem. In fact, it can actually be a positive force in our lives. It provides us with novelty, challenges, and opportunities for growth. Chronic stress, however, has a profoundly negative effect on health and is a common trigger for Meniere's disease episodes. It is essential to try to eliminate stress and reduce anxiety.

I have struggled with anxiety for most of my life, long before I had ever heard of Meniere's disease. It reached a tipping point when, at 18 years old, my best friend suddenly passed away. From that point forward, I had to take medication to control my anxiety and panic attacks. This went on for years. The medication helped me deal with the symptoms of my anxiety, but I never dealt with the underlying issues that were causing the symptoms. Eventually, I started seeing a therapist to try to understand and address the root cause of my anxiety. Later on, this same therapist was crucial in helping me process the chaos that came with my Meniere's diagnosis. Therapy helped me considerably, but it was not until much later that I discovered meditation.

Learning how to meditate, and practicing regularly, was by far the most powerful tool I have ever found for dealing with my anxiety and stress. My whole demeanor and personality began to transform. I suddenly found myself less bothered by the little things. And when bigger issues did inevitably arise, I was less anxious, and the anxiety lasted for a much shorter period of time. After a while, I realized for the first time in nearly six years that maybe I would be okay without medication. With my doctor's blessing, I started to wean myself off and soon found myself no longer dependent on the anti-anxiety meds. I stood on my own two feet again and the world did not come crashing down around me. Without meditation, I don't know if I ever would have gotten to that point. When I was eventually diagnosed with Meniere's disease, my meditation practice became a powerful force in my recovery.

What is Meditation?

The human brain is the most powerful information processing "machine" in the known universe and we're born without an instruction manual. It's amazing to me that Western culture doesn't take more of an interest in learning how to manage the mind. But learning to master your thoughts is an incredibly valuable skill to have in life. For many people, their thoughts and mental chatter seem to be outside of their control; a chaotic whirlwind of reminders, insights, negative self-talk and random bits of narrative. Most people don't even realize that it's possible to develop control over your mind and your thoughts.

Simply put, meditation is a practice of quieting the mind. In many Eastern traditions, meditation is a tool for spiritual development, as well. But for treating Meniere's disease, stress reduction is our goal, not spiritual growth.

Meditation has a powerful effect on the body and mind. In the short term, it triggers a relaxation response that calms the nervous system and, as a result, the body and mind. It causes an immediate reduction of stress, as well. For treating Meniere's disease, this alone would be enough, but it doesn't end there. It's the long-term effects that are the most desirable. Your overall level of stress will start to go down while your ability to cope with stress becomes stronger. Your ability to focus and concentrate will improve. When stress does occur, you will be able to center and calm yourself much more quickly. You will react less and respond more. The ability to quiet your mind will allow you to fall asleep faster and more easily. All of these benefits are priceless and will drastically reduce the time it takes you to get your symptoms under control.

How to Meditate

There are many different approaches to meditation. Some are easier than others, but all of them require regular daily practice to be effective. In my experience, the best way to have success with meditation is to incorporate it into your daily routine. Set aside the same small block of time every day. When building any new habit, adding it to your routine will help to make it stick. It also helps to set an attainable starting goal; a mere 5-10 minutes a day is perfect. If you try to do it for longer than that initially, you may get frustrated and decide to give up before getting any real benefit. Once you have successfully adopted the habit, you can gradually increase the time. Personally, I meditate for 20-30 minutes every day.

Most approaches to meditation involve focusing your attention on a single point of awareness. Mantra meditation is a perfect example of this. A mantra is simply a word, phrase, or sound. By focusing your mind on a mentally repeated mantra, other thoughts are quieted.

At first glance, meditation seems easy, but most people quickly find that it is much more difficult in practice. The most important thing to understand is this: there is no such thing as failure when it comes to meditation. In the beginning, you may find it very difficult to focus. Thoughts will pop in at random and distract you. This is perfectly normal. Anytime you become aware of these other thoughts, just gently bring your focus back. With time and practice, you will find it gets easier and easier.

The breath plays an important role in mediation, as well. Stress causes our breathing to become shallow and constricted, filling only a small portion of our lungs with oxygen. When you are stressed, it's important to take deep breaths into your diaphragm. The diaphragm is the muscle in your abdomen that controls your lungs. Feel your stomach expand as you take slow, deep, steady breaths. It will cause your nervous system to calm down and will start to relax you. With meditation, conscious control of your breath is an important goal. Our breath and body are intimately connected. When your breathing is calm and controlled, your body will be, as well.

Technique #1 - Stomach Breathing Meditation

Stomach breathing is a simple and powerful approach to meditation. For beginners, it's a great way to get started. It can be done while sitting or lying down. Turn the lights off and get comfortable. Set a timer for 5-10 minutes and turn your phone off or on silent to avoid distractions. Close your eyes and start taking slow deep breaths into your diaphragm. Consciously relax your muscles, starting with your feet and working your way up to your head. As you continue to breathe, focus your mind on the physical sensations of your abdomen. Feel the movement of the muscles as they expand and contract. Continue until your timer goes off. If you catch your thoughts drifting away from your stomach, gently guide your focus back. You will find that this happens less and less over time.

Technique #2 - Counting Breath Meditation

This is another great technique for beginners. It can

be done sitting or lying down. Set a timer for 5-10 minutes and make sure you will not be distracted. Turn the lights off and get comfortable. Again, consciously relax your muscles, starting with your feet and working your way up to your head.

With each inhale, hold your mind completely blank. As you exhale, count the breath (in your mind) throughout the whole exhale.

It goes like this: inhale (mind blank), exhale (ooooonnnnnnnneeeeee), inhale (mind blank), exhale (ttttttttwwwwwwwoooooooooo), inhale (mind blank), exhale (tttttthhhhhrrrrreeeeeee), and so on. Keep going until you count your 10th exhale, and then start over back at one. Repeat until your timer goes off. If you catch your mind drifting, gently bring it back to the exercise and start the count back at one.

Technique #3 - Mantra Meditation

Mantra meditation has become very popular worldwide as a result of the Transcendental Meditation movement, also known as TM. TM is taught through a paid course, where an instructor gives a private mantra to the student. The technique is taught and the student practices. Many people report that having an instructor and having to pay for classes helps to keep them accountable, and, as a result, the habit sticks. It is not necessary, however, to pay for TM classes. Mantra meditation can be done on your own. First though, you have to select a mantra. You can use "Om" if you'd like, but really any word will do. Sometimes I use "infinity" as a mantra. Whatever word you choose, its purpose is to act as a point of focus for your mind.

Like the previous two techniques, it can be done sitting comfortably or lying down. Set a timer and make sure you will not be distracted. Close your eyes and consciously relax your muscles, starting with your feet and working your way up to your head. Start to breathe deeply into your diaphragm. After each breath, mentally repeat your mantra. Focus your attention on the mantra and hold your mind clear as you take each breath. If you find your thoughts drifting, that's okay. Just gently bring your focus back to the mantra. Repeat this until your timer goes off.

Technique #4 - Tinnitus Meditation

Tinnitus is one of the most frustrating symptoms of Meniere's disease. It's not generally as debilitating as vertigo, but it's usually present even if you get your other symptoms under control. The constant ringing and buzzing can drive you crazy. I've found that meditation is extremely helpful in learning to manage tinnitus. The better you are at controlling your thoughts, the better you are at placing your attention elsewhere. However, while meditating I stumbled upon something interesting. While most techniques for managing tinnitus involve learning to ignore it, a better approach is to focus on it intentionally.

People are bothered by tinnitus the most when they are trying to ignore it, but can't, no matter how hard they try. It occurred to me one day, instead of trying to block it out, why not face it head on? Meditation involves concentrating our focus on a single point of awareness, so why not focus on the ringing? I found that, much to my surprise, by choosing to focus intensely on the sound, it was much easier to ignore later on. It seemed to lose its power over me. It may seem counterintuitive, but it works amazingly well. Stress often can make your tinnitus worse, so any practice that combines improving tinnitus and meditation is a winning combination in my book.

The technique, like the others, is fairly simple. It can be done sitting or lying down. Get comfortable and set a timer for 5-10 minutes. Make sure you will not be distracted, especially by other sounds. You need silence for this exercise. Close your eyes and take a couple of deep breaths. Consciously relax all of your muscles, starting with your feet and working your way up to your head. Next, focus your entire attention on the sound of your tinnitus. For the first several minutes, just maintain this focus. If you find your mind drifting, gently bring it back to the sound of your tinnitus. Sound can be a powerful tool to focus your awareness into a single point. Hopefully, you will find yourself deeply relaxing into a meditative state. See if you can find variations in the sound. If you listen carefully, you may find there are multiple tones or noises. Explore this with a mindset of curiosity.

Next, while still focusing on the sound, imagine that there is a large volume knob in front of you that controls the volume of the sound. Imagine yourself playing with the volume knob, turning it up and down. You may be as surprised as I was to find that the volume of the sound can be affected. Sometimes I imagine a large on/off switch, as well, and mentally flip it up and down. Now imagine that there is a second knob right next to the volume, which controls the tone of the sound. Imagine yourself turning this knob, too. I was amazed to find that I can temporarily lower and raise the frequency of the tones of my tinnitus by doing this. Continue to focus on the sound until your timer goes off.

I've noticed that if I catch my mind drifting from the sound of my tinnitus, for that brief bit of time, my tinnitus wasn't bothering me at all. Like all meditation though, it will take practice. There are not enough good techniques for managing tinnitus. I hope this practice can help you as much as it has helped me.

Counseling and Support Groups

Even the strongest of personal support networks may not be enough to support your needs. Having Meniere's disease can be a traumatic experience. The hopeless despair and seemingly endless suffering is enough to leave a deep emotional scar on the toughest of us. Many doctors seem to only compound the fear, leaving us worse for wear. The resulting trauma needs to be addressed.

I have seen and felt the damage first-hand that unresolved trauma can cause. I've witnessed the chaos and devastation that can manifest years, even decades, after the trauma occurred. Fortunately, there are several good ways to address this, sooner rather than later.

When I was 18, after my best friend had died, I suddenly became a very anxious person. As the years went on, it only got worse, and I became an angry person, as well. I had never properly grieved and processed the death of my friend. The emotions, still bottled up inside of me, would pour out through the cracks in my armor and leave a path of destruction in their wake. But at the time I didn't understand. It wasn't until much later, in therapy, that the connection between the trauma and my anxiety became clear.

Counseling, or "talk therapy," can be a cathartic and an overwhelmingly positive experience when at its best. Similar to finding the right doctor, you'll need to find the right therapist. There are several therapeutic styles to choose from. For me personally, a type of therapy called Cognitive Behavioral Therapy worked best. I suspect, however, that my success has had more to do with my actual therapist than the type of therapy. When I was diagnosed with Meniere's disease, I had already been with my therapist for a while, working through my anxiety. His personality really seemed to mesh with mine, and he was always positive, encouraging, and hopeful.

Like most people, he had never heard of Meniere's disease but took the time to listen and learn about it. When I was diagnosed, he helped me to stay calm and in the moment while it felt like my world was falling apart. He helped me process the turmoil and crazy mishmash of emotions I felt. And when I finally found the best doctor to treat my Meniere's disease, the one who set me on the right path, I was able to actually hear what he had to say. My therapist had kept me grounded enough to listen and be open to new information. I've been with the same therapist for eight years now. If you can find a therapist you trust, it can be a powerfully rewarding experience and one that I can't recommend enough.

If counseling doesn't fit into your budget, you still have options. Support groups can be a great choice. The Vestibular Disorders Association website features a support group directory (Vestibular.org/finding-help-support/support-directory). If you search by location, you may find support group meetings close to where you live. If not, there are vibrant support group communities online. Having a place to openly vent frustrations, celebrate successes, and communicate with others in the same situation can be extremely helpful.

Support group communities exist in several locations. There are several forums and message boards on the internet solely devoted to Meniere's disease. Additionally, there are many great support groups on Facebook. Facebook's ability to create groups around a central topic is a great platform for Meniere's disease support groups. There are a good number of them, some with thousands of highly active and supportive members. Questions are generally answered very quickly and by a large number of people.

You can find the Facebook group I run here: Facebook.com/groups/MenieresDiseaseSupportGroup/. But with a simple search for Meniere's disease on Facebook, you will find a handful of other groups. A list of online support communities can be found in the resources section in the back of the book.

If you find, however, that spending time in these communities is bringing you down, I suggest you avoid them for a while. Some of the groups can have a "misery loves company" kind of feel to them at times. If a group is putting a damper on your mood, it's better to explore other, more positive avenues. There is always so much hope. Never forget that.

Gratitude and Mindset

When your suffering is at its worst, it's incredibly hard to be grateful for anything. We simply aren't wired to naturally have gratitude when times are tough. People have a tendency to hone in the cause of their pain with a focus and intensity rarely seen elsewhere in their lives. But it's completely possible to retrain your brain to focus on, and find the good in, every situation. No matter where you are in terms of managing your Meniere's symptoms, the lifestyle and mindset advantages of a gratitude practice are substantial. Like meditation, successfully adopting a gratitude practice takes time, but the payoff is huge and it's worth the effort.

Practicing gratitude will help you stay positive and hopeful more often. In the framework of treating Meniere's disease, it will shift your focus away from the suffering and symptoms of your worst days, to the incredible peace and exhilaration of your good days. Even if you are having a difficult time managing your symptoms, changing your frame of mind with a gratitude practice can make all the difference. It reveals the silver lining, always hidden just behind the veil of your suffering. It allows you to truly enjoy the good days. And when the storm does come, you will endure, knowing in your heart that this too shall pass, that everything will be okay. Most importantly, it's within your power to make this change. It might take a bit of creativity at first, but no matter how bad things may seem, you can start this practice immediately.

My favorite approach to starting a gratitude practice is to first get a journal or notepad, separate from the one you use to track your lifestyle. The practice itself is extremely simple. Every day, make a list of five to ten things you are grateful for. Try to come up with five to ten new things each day.

At first, you will think of the obvious examples, like family, friends, and other loved ones. As you go on though, you will have to really stretch your mind to fill out your list. You might get stuck; that's okay. Keep at it until you have a list of five to ten things.

Get creative with it! For example, if you are at home recovering from a vertigo attack, perhaps you are getting time to spend with your spouse that you wouldn't have otherwise. If your symptoms are under control but you are having a bit of brain fog, you can be grateful for a day without vertigo. It's incredibly difficult to remain in a bad mood after focusing my brain so intensely on coming up with a whole list of things I'm grateful for.

Another interesting approach to gratitude is a product called the Five Minute Journal (FiveMinuteJournal.com). It's a beautifully designed physical journal that takes only five minutes to complete in the morning and in the evening with daily prompts. It directs you to focus on the positive right as you wake up, and then to reflect back on your day right before you go to bed. They also sell it as an app for your smart phone.

The advantage of this system is its simplicity and ease of adoption. It's incredibly easy to add into your daily routine. Megan leaves hers on her nightstand and quickly fills it out each morning and night. It is a great approach to easily add gratitude into your daily routine.

The One Minute
Gratitude Breathing Exercise

The following is a technique that was invented by Heartmath, an organization that studies the connection between the heart and the brain (Heartmath.com). They have done some really innovative research and designed incredibly effective products.

The technique is officially called "Quick Coherence® Technique." According to Heartmath, it was designed to help you "find a feeling of ease and inner harmony that's reflected in more balanced heart rhythms, facilitating brain function and access to higher intelligence." I have had powerful results with this technique and generally feel a deep sense of peace and gratitude afterward. It can cause an immediate shift in your mindset and is a valuable tool in your Meniere's toolkit.

From Heartmath:

"**Step 1:** Focus your attention in the area of the heart. Imagine your breath is flowing in and out of your heart or chest area, breathing a little slower and deeper than usual.

Suggestion: Inhale 5 seconds, exhale 5 seconds (or whatever rhythm is comfortable)

Step 2: Make a sincere attempt to experience a regenerative feeling such as appreciation or care for someone or something in your life.

Suggestion: Try to re-experience the feeling you have for someone you love, a pet, a special place, an accomplishment, etc. or focus on a feeling of calm or ease."

You can stop after a minute or continue for as long as you'd like.

Mentally Overcoming Setbacks and Difficult Days

The one thing I know with absolute certainty is that nothing stays the same forever. Change is the constant we can always rely on. It's a good thing, too. Without change, we would lack the perspective to understand good and bad; our experiences would simply be indifferent.

We can only ever truly appreciate a beautiful experience by first knowing hardship, and what it means to suffer. Understanding is found in the contrast.

With a condition as unpredictable as Meniere's disease, change can often come as a wave of relief or a flood of hardship. If you have been able to gain some control over your symptoms, change can be an unwelcomed visitor.

There is nothing more frustrating than facing a setback after making progress in your treatment and recovery. It can rob you of precious hope and leave you feeling crushed. But it doesn't have to be this way. No matter how dark the hole you find yourself in, you still have the power to make choices.

Marcus Aurelius, the last great Roman Emperor and a Stoic Philosopher, had a profound view on the nature of change: "The universe is change; our life is what our thoughts make it." This is a remarkable insight made in the second century AD, and yet, still rings as true today as it did nearly 1,850 years ago. There is a considerable amount of practical knowledge to be learned from the great Stoics of history.

When facing a setback or difficult day, sometimes the best choice is to simply interpret your situation differently. The Stoic philosophers believed that events themselves were inherently meaningless. That it's the story we tell ourselves afterward about what the event means that categorizes it as "good" or "bad."

Setbacks can come in all shapes and sizes. If you find yourself having a tough time, unable to get anything done or meet your responsibilities, don't feel guilty or be too hard on yourself.

When you are actively suffering, whether from Meniere's disease or otherwise, it can be hard to see anything but pain. Sometimes, simply acknowledging the pain can be enough:

- Give yourself permission to not feel well
- Give yourself permission to have a bad day
- Give yourself permission to rest, and let your body heal

It's a subtle shift in perspective, but it can make all the difference. Everyone will experience setbacks at one point or another, and the more you can roll with the punches, the quicker you will bounce back, every time. If your body needs to heal, let it heal. Feed it the things it needs to become whole. Let yourself rest knowing that when this setback inevitably passes, you will truly appreciate the good days that follow. There is never shame in being sick, and no matter how bad things may seem in the moment, you will make progress again.

Physical Stress Relief

So far, most of this section has focused on strategies for managing your mind. Yet managing and maintaining your body is also crucially important when trying to eliminate stress. Stress often finds its way into our physical bodies as muscle tension, aches and pains, and general discomfort. You'll find that taking care of your body in a way that reduces physical stress will benefit you mentally and emotionally, as well. The mind and body are intimately connected. Taking a whole body, or holistic, approach to your health is a good way to set yourself up to fight off your Meniere's symptoms effectively.

Massage

Massage, in all its forms, may seem like a luxury, but it is also a powerful tool for healing. An experienced masseuse can relieve tense and knotted muscles throughout the whole body. Our bodies tend to store anxiety, stress, emotional pain, and fear as physical tension in the body. It's an insidious type of tension, too. We don't even realize the toll it takes on us until it's gotten so bad that we feel it as pain. Getting a professional massage, once a month, has had a transformative effect on my stress level. It is mind boggling how much tension accumulates in my muscles over the course of a single month. If you can afford it, getting a massage, even if it's only once every couple of months, can be extremely effective for dealing with stress.

If a professional massage is not in the budget, there are other less expensive ways of managing physical stress. My personal favorite happens to be the cheapest possible option: the lacrosse ball. You can find them at any sporting goods store for a couple of dollars and they can be a life saver. You can use them to massage and work the tension out of most of the muscles in your body. Generally, I will lie on my back with the lacrosse ball under my shoulder blades and slowly work the ball around my back and shoulder muscles. It works really well on sore feet, too. Be gentle at first and slowly add pressure as needed.

Acupuncture

Acupuncture is one of the main components of Traditional Chinese Medicine (TCM) and is a practice that dates back thousands of years. To understand acupuncture, you must first understand that TCM believes that the body contains a system of energy flow pathways called meridians. Hundreds of points, known as meridian points, have been identified along these pathways that have a direct effect on the body. The energy that flows through the meridian pathways is known as Qi (pronounced chi). TCM follows the thinking that our health is closely tied to the free flow of Qi and that blockages result in health problems. An acupuncturist places long, thin needles into various meridian points to clear these blockages.

If it all sounds very esoteric, I highly encourage you to keep an open mind. In the last decade, Western culture has seen a massive rise in the popularity of acupuncture as a means to treat a wide variety of ailments, illnesses, and pain. Many hospitals now offer therapeutic acupuncture as an accompaniment to pharmaceutical and traditional medical approaches. Many Meniere's patients often report a reduction in symptoms following a series of acupuncture sessions. At the very least, I encourage you to try it before you make a judgment. TCM has existed for far longer than our Western, science-based medicine. Its longevity is a testament to its efficacy.

When I was first diagnosed, I immediately started seeing an acupuncturist. It definitely lessened my vertigo. Some people find immediate relief from their symptoms while, for others, it may take several sessions. It is important to find an experienced acupuncturist for the best chance of success. A quick Google search should reveal acupuncturists in your area. Call and talk to them, and don't be afraid to ask questions. Explain your Meniere's disease and your symptoms, and find out if they are familiar with it.

Surprisingly, my acupuncturist had treated Meniere's patients before, as well as patients with other causes of vertigo and tinnitus.

Saunas

Saunas are another fantastic tool for stress reduction and have the added benefit of increasing your overall capacity for dealing with stress. Also, the heat of the sauna will quickly relax sore and stiff muscles. Twenty minutes in the sauna should be more than enough to work up a good sweat. I find after a sauna I feel incredibly relaxed and refreshed. For me, there's nothing like hopping in the sauna after a good workout.

In terms of treating Meniere's disease, the sweat decreases fluid retention much in the same way a diuretic does. I've found that saunas have helped to reduce the feeling of pressure in my ears. Remember to stay hydrated, though. Make sure to drink plenty of water before you start and after you finish.

Journaling and Stress

Stress is, without question, one of the most common triggers of Meniere's episodes and symptoms. This is most likely due to the toll stress can take on your immune system. Writing in your journal can help to decrease your stress levels in several important ways.

First and foremost, writing down your fears, stresses, and anxieties makes them concrete. When they remain undefined, freely floating around in your mind, they can overwhelm you and cause undue stress. Until your fears are made clear, they often appear to be much larger than they actually are. It's the uncertainty that drives your anxiety. The act of writing organizes your thoughts into a clear and understandable form. Keep track of your stress levels as well as stressful events in your journal, the same way you keep track of your diet. It will help you to identify and reduce the stress-based triggers of your symptoms.

Reducing your fear can also help to reduce your stress. In his best-selling book, *The Four Hour Workweek*, author and human performance guru Tim Ferriss describes his approach to conquering fear. "To do or not to do? To try or not to try? Most people will vote no, whether they consider themselves brave or not. Uncertainty and the prospect of failure can be very scary noises in the shadows. Most people will choose unhappiness over uncertainty."

Tim argues that by clearly defining your fear in explicit detail, you can reach your goals, achieve your dreams, and reduce your stress. If you find yourself stressed out and afraid to take action, Tim offers up a simple exercise to try called Fear Setting.

In your journal, divide a page into three columns.

In the first column, write down everything that

could possibly go wrong if you were to take the action you're considering. Be explicit. Define the worst possible scenario in as much detail as possible.

In the second column, list all the ways you can prevent each item in the first column from happening. What steps can you take ahead of time to eliminate negative outcomes?

Finally in the third column, describe how you could recover from each scenario you described in the first column. If your worst fears came true, how could you bounce back? Could you turn it to your advantage? At the very least, describe how you could move forward with your life.

To take it a step further, an interesting twist on this exercise is to face your fear with an expectation of failure. Assume that everything will go wrong and decide what your next move will be. Given these new circumstances, what steps can you take to make sure you will still live a life of satisfaction and purpose? Make a concrete plan of what you will do after it inevitably blows up in your face.

If you take this approach, you will always have a positive outcome. If nothing goes wrong, then you will have far exceeded your expectations. Otherwise, everything will have gone according to plan and you will know exactly what to do next. It's an excellent strategy to reduce stress.

Reducing your stress levels will also help you to get

better sleep. Like stress, sleep deprivation can trigger your symptoms in a big way. Get enough high-quality sleep, and your health will start to improve. In the next section, I will show you how reduce your symptoms by getting better sleep, starting tonight.

SLEEP

"Sleep is that golden chain that ties health and our bodies together." – Thomas Dekker

Without sleep, it can all break down so quickly. After only a few restless nights, I start to come apart at the seams. The screaming bells in my ears make it impossible to hear myself think. My stress levels peak. The ear pressure builds, and the dizziness begins. Sleep is so important and is often an overlooked aspect of treating Meniere's disease.

Sleep is so many things. It can be one of the greatest simple pleasures in life. It can be a frustrating nuisance that keeps us from our life's work. It can be a blissful peace or a restless nightmare. Whatever sleep may be to you, there's no question that it's an absolutely necessary component of health.

Sleep science and research have progressed considerably over the last several years. Our understanding has evolved, but the vast majority of us continue to be overworked, overstressed, and sleep deprived. It's hard to believe that sleep could be the answer to the question of health; it seems too easy. But so often in life, it's the little things that make the biggest difference.

Getting plenty of high-quality sleep is one of the most powerful tools in your arsenal against Meniere's disease. Get enough good sleep, and you'll experience a powerful healing effect across all of your other treatment efforts. Get too little, though, and your health will crumble while symptoms get worse and worse.

Basic Sleep Science

Even though we all share the need to sleep, trying to explain exactly what sleep is can be challenging. It's like trying to explain the meaning of life. But we don't need to understand what sleep is to know its effect on human health. It's a good idea, however, to first get a basic understanding of sleep science so you can learn how to improve.

In his book *Sleep Smarter*, Shawn Stevenson writes, "Generally, being awake is catabolic (breaks you down) and sleep is anabolic (builds you up). Sleep is known to be an elevated anabolic state, heightening the growth and rejuvenation of the immune, skeletal, and muscular systems... High-quality sleep fortifies your immune system, balances your hormones, boosts your metabolism, increases physical energy and improves the function of your brain." The average person will never reach their full potential without getting enough quality sleep. For someone suffering from Meniere's disease, improving your sleep is a crucial starting point and necessary part of improving your health. If you don't factor the quality of your sleep into your treatment, you will put yourself at a major disadvantage.

Throughout the night, the nature of sleep changes in a regular and predictable way. There are several phases of sleep, each serving a different purpose, that occur in repeating 90-minute cycles. Each 90-minute cycle includes a period of physiologically restorative deep sleep, a transition to lighter sleep, and psychologically restorative REM (Rapid Eye Movement) sleep, where our minds are highly active and dreaming occurs. People typically sleep for a total of four to six, 90-minute sleep cycles each night, for a total of 6-9 hours of sleep.

If you find that you often feel tired when you wake up after a full night of sleep, try this simple trick. Set your alarm to wake you after 7.5 hours or 9 hours of sleep, instead of the "standard 8 hours." This corresponds to either five or six 90-minute sleep cycles. If you wake up in the middle of a sleep cycle, you may be groggier than usual. This simple trick can be hugely helpful in having more energy in the morning. When you're dealing with Meniere's symptoms, the more energy you have in the morning, the better your chances of having a successful day. It's hard to be motivated to do anything when you wake up feeling brain fogged and tired, on top of your other symptoms.

Sleep Deprivation

Even for a healthy adult, the effects of sleep deprivation are debilitating. For someone with Meniere's disease, sleep deprivation can prevent all progress in your treatment. It's important to understand that our body does not treat sleep like a bank. You can't save up sleep and try to go for days without it. You also can't "overdraft" without consequences, getting less sleep during the week and expecting just to make it up on the weekends. To receive the benefits that sleep can provide for your health, you have to make an effort to get quality sleep as much as possible. If you don't, you will end up paying the price, whether you realize it or not.

There are a wide variety of damaging effects that result from a chronic lack of sleep. In the short term, sleep deprivation will reduce your cognitive performance and alertness, beginning even after just one night of poor sleep. Sleep deprivation will affect your memory, as well. Brain fog and cognitive impairment are already an unfortunate part of life for a Meniere's disease sufferer. Getting adequate sleep will reduce its impact. Lack of sleep can also decrease your ability to handle stress and increase your overall stress load. It will depress your immune system and can increase levels of inflammation throughout the body.

In the long term, the effects of chronic sleep deprivation are even worse. They include high blood pressure, higher risk of heart attack and heart failure, higher risk of stroke, obesity, mental health issues such as anxiety disorders and depression, attention disorders such as ADD, a decrease in emotional intelligence, and an overall decrease in quality of life.

I find that when I don't get enough sleep for several days in a row, my health starts to break down and my Meniere's symptoms flare up. Sleep deprivation causes a terrible cascade of negative consequences that can all be avoided by simply taking steps to improve the quality of your sleep.

Sleep Hygiene

Now that you have a basic understanding, the best strategy is to optimize the quality of your sleep as much as possible. You may be getting an adequate amount of sleep, but that doesn't mean that you're getting quality sleep. The difference is profound. There are many effective techniques that will all contribute towards getting you the best night sleep possible.

Turn Off All of Your Screens

For better or worse, bright backlit screens have come

to dominate our lives. Our smartphones, tablets, laptops, and TVs have become the centerpieces of our increasingly interconnected world. Though they enhance our lives in numerous ways, they disrupt the quality of our sleep.

Our bodies maintain an internal day/night cycle known as the circadian rhythm. During the day, sunlight triggers our bodies to secrete day time hormones. (Getting 10-30 minutes of sunlight first thing in the morning is another way to increase your energy in the morning.) At night, in the absence of sunlight, our brains secrete a hormone called melatonin. Melatonin lets our bodies know that it's night and time to get ready to go to sleep. Unfortunately, the bright blue light emitted from our various screens causes our brain to reduce the production of melatonin. Watching TV or reading on your iPad before bed can make it harder to fall asleep and degrades the quality of your sleep.

To avoid this pitfall, you have several options. The best option is also the simplest: turn off all backlit screens 90 minutes before bedtime. Read a book (a paper book, not an eBook) instead or spend time with loved ones. This is your best way to ensure a good night's sleep.

If this isn't possible, you still have some additional choices. The first is to get a pair of glasses that block the blue light spectrum. You can find blue light blocking glasses on Amazon.com for very cheap, or you can opt for the pricier, yet more stylish Blublocker brand sunglasses. They both work the same. The blue light spectrum emitted from our devices mimics sunlight and shuts down melatonin production. Wearing these glasses will block this spectrum of light and protect the quality of your sleep.

The final option is a software option for your smartphone, tablet, or laptop. There are several great apps for your computer and mobile devices that will dim the screen and apply a red tinted filter that turns off most of the blue light spectrum. Use F.Lux for laptops and computers and Twilight for Andriod devices. Unfortunately, there are currently no apps for Apple IOS devices that do this.

Set Up Your Bedroom for the
Best Possible Sleep

There are several simple changes you can make to your bedroom environment to immediately improve the quality of your sleep. The first has to with light. If you have a lot of ambient light coming into your bedroom from nightlights, cable boxes, alarm clocks, street lights outside, or anywhere else, it can disrupt the quality of your sleep. The best strategy is to make your room as dark as possible. You can find blackout curtains at most department stores. Also, cover every source of light in your bedroom, no matter how small. Ideally, you want your room to be pitch black. This is something that you can do right now to improve the quality of your sleep. A simpler solution is to wear a sleep mask that covers your eyes. It works just as well but may not be as comfortable for some people. I have a hard time falling asleep with an eye mask.

The next variable is room temperature. Studies have shown that we get the best sleep when the temperature in the room is between 60 and 68 degrees Fahrenheit. It's much cooler than you would expect and has to do with a bodily process called thermoregulation. Again Shawn Stevenson explains: "When it's time for your body to rest, there is an automatic drop in your core body temperature to help initiate sleep. If the temperature in your environment stays too high, then it can be a bit of a physiological challenge for your body to get into the ideal state for restful sleep." If the temperature is much warmer or cooler than the optimum range, it might impact your sleep. Wearing socks is a good option if your feet get cold at this temperature. I keep my thermostat at 68 degrees at night with a ceiling fan on low.

The sound of your environment also has a direct effect on your sleep. For a Meniere's patient, this presents an interesting set of challenges. Under normal circumstances, it's important to have a silent sleep environment. Even a small noise can stir you awake;

whether you remember it the next morning or not is irrelevant. It disrupts your sleep cycles and lowers your quality of sleep. The challenge here is that tinnitus is typically much worse and more noticeable in silence. There are several good ways to overcome this. You can either attempt to mask the noise of your tinnitus, drowning it out with relaxing background noise, or use meditative techniques.

Tinnitus and Sleep

Your success in masking the sound of your tinnitus depends entirely on your level of hearing. If you have suffered any degree of hearing loss, this method may not work as well. If you have already lost your hearing entirely, this method won't work at all. So assuming you still have some or all of your hearing left, there are various ways to add background noise to your bedroom to drown out your tinnitus. The first is a white noise machine. White noise is essentially a whooshing static sound that is played continually. Many people find white noise to be a pleasant and relaxing sound. There are many different white noise machines available.

A better alternative to a white noise machine is a sound therapy machine. Sound therapy machines are typically small alarm clock sized devices that play a wide range of soothing sounds that I find much more desirable than white noise. You can, however, also use your cell phone as a sound machine. If you have a smartphone, there are hundreds of apps that generate all different types of ambient background noise. You can enhance this system by connecting your phone to a portable Bluetooth speaker. I prefer this option because there are so many different sounds to choose from. You can keep trying different apps until you find the perfect sound that masks your tinnitus and allows you to fall asleep. The sound of a "babbling brook" generally does it for me.

If masking the sound of your tinnitus is not an option, meditative techniques are the way to go. In the chapter on Stress and Mental Well-being, I described a technique called the tinnitus meditation. In addition to being a great way to reduce the impact of tinnitus, it's an incredibly powerful tool for falling asleep.

Use this simplified version of the tinnitus meditation to fall asleep quickly:

As you lay down to go to sleep, get comfortable, close your eyes, and take a couple of deep breaths into your diaphragm (abdomen). Consciously relax your whole body, starting with your feet, working your way up to your head. Once your body is relaxed, focus your entire attention on the sound of your tinnitus. If you find your mind drifting, gently bring it back to the sound. Keep your mind focused on the sound and you will slowly find yourself drifting off to sleep.

I have had tremendous success with this method, even with earplugs in. Without this technique, sleeping with earplugs would be impossible for me. The silence of wearing earplugs causes the volume of my tinnitus to increase substantially, but with this technique it doesn't matter. I fall right to sleep.

Falling Asleep

When it comes to falling asleep, I find people generally tend to fall into two basic categories: those who can with no effort at all and those who can't. This section is written for the latter; the people who, like me, struggle to fall asleep far more often than not. To get quality sleep, you obviously need to fall asleep first. Fighting to fall asleep is an unnecessary source of stress for many people.

No matter how tired I am, as soon as my head hits the pillow, my brain decides to fire on all cylinders. My thoughts seem to race off ahead of me, dictating my schedule for tomorrow, reviewing everything that happened today, and coming up with new ideas. Sometimes, I treasure the clarity that comes at this moment. But more often it's quickly followed by the realization that I won't be falling asleep anytime soon. This is how our minds tend to function during the day, as well, but we are usually way too distracted to realize that it's happening. With the constant barrage of external stimuli we face all day long, we rarely pay attention to the nature of our thoughts. But once we are comfortable in our beds, where most of the sensory input is gone, we are left alone with our thoughts, undistracted. I know how frustrating it can be when it feels like you just can't stop thinking. Over the years, I have found several techniques that work really well to fall asleep quickly and painlessly.

The Mind Dump:

When you are trying to fall asleep, a lot of the mental chatter stems from trying to juggle a list of things to remember. It can be especially bad when you are trying to fall asleep and suddenly have an idea. The "AHA" moment that comes with a new idea can trigger a dopamine release, keeping you awake. Not to mention that you probably will want to remember the idea. No matter what thoughts are swirling around in your mind, the act of putting them down on paper before you get in bed can make all the difference.

Writing in your journal before you go to sleep is the perfect solution. Take a few minutes to sit down and perform what I like to call a mind dump. Whatever you find yourself thinking about, just write it all down, it's as simple as that. You will find that you can fall asleep afterward much more easily with your thoughts and ideas safely backed up in hardcopy. Sleep has a strange way of robbing us of the thoughts we have as we are drifting off, no matter how sure we are that we will remember them in the morning. Most people never do. If you find that you still have persistent thoughts and ideas after your mind dump, turn the light back on and write down anything else you might have missed.

Relaxation Techniques

One of the most useful things I discovered over the years is that it's often physical tension that prevents us from falling asleep. As you fall asleep, your body and brain go through a series of changes. Your brainwaves slow down and your body starts to physically relax. I've found that you can hack this process by consciously relaxing your body first. Once your body is completely relaxed, you will likely find yourself drifting off to sleep. It's amazing how much physical tension we can hold in our muscles without realizing it. When you focus intensely on relaxing muscle groups throughout your body, you will start to notice it. Once you release the tension, your body can quickly drop into sleep.

To implement this, I developed a routine I call the "Elevator Method" for falling asleep. It combines physical muscle relaxation, breathing techniques, and visualization. It is extremely effective and simple to perform.

The Elevator Method

The first step is to lie down and get completely comfortable. Take several deep breaths into your diaphragm. Consciously relax your entire body and go limp like a ragdoll. Next, focus on individual muscle groups, one at a time, relaxing each as much as possible. Let all the tension go as you work through your body. Start with your feet and your toes; let the muscles go completely limp. Move up to your legs and your butt, let all the tension go. Continue on to your stomach and your lower back, then your chest and upper back, your shoulders and your arms, your hands and your fingers, your neck and your throat, and finally, your head and your face.

Once your muscles are completely relaxed, clear your mind with 5 deep counting breaths. On each slow inhale, hold your mind completely clear. As you exhale, count the breath in your mind. Repeat this until you count 5 breaths.

Finally, imagine the bed is inside an elevator, descending deep underground with the elevator doors still open. Imagine the elevator shaft is made of dirt, and as you descend down, imagine you can see the dirt walls appearing to move up as you sink deeper and deeper down the elevator shaft. Try to feel this sense of sinking with your entire body. You may be surprised to find you actually feel like the bed is sinking down beneath you. Hold this in your imagination for as long as you can. Feel the bed sinking, down and down and down. Deeper and deeper down.

By this point, you should be on the verge of falling asleep, or at the very least, deeply relaxed. This technique becomes more effective the more often you practice it. Your body will start to associate the routine with falling asleep.

Initially, it can help to have someone else guide you through this practice. The first time I guided Megan through this routine, she was asleep before I finished. She had been tossing and turning for over an hour, unable to sleep. I hope it works for you as well as it has worked for us.

Binaural Beats

Binaural beats are specially engineered sounds that produce changes in your brain state and are a safe and effective way to induce sleep. The technology itself is simple to use but a little difficult to understand. It works like this: by listening to a single tone in one ear, say 500Hz, and a slightly different tone in the other ear, say 504Hz, the difference of 4Hz happens to be the same frequency as Theta brain waves. Through a process called entrainment, your brain will start producing more Theta brainwaves simply by listening to the binaural beat through headphones (it won't work otherwise). A Theta dominant brain state usually occurs during light sleep and deep meditation.

Binaural beats can be used to induce meditative states, alert states, and creative states, as well. But by syncing your brain with the brainwaves that correspond with sleep, such as Theta and Delta, you can fall asleep very quickly. To work effectively, binaural beats must be listened to through headphones. If you have lost your hearing in one or both ears, binaural beats, unfortunately, will not work for you.

There are many choices available if you would like to explore binaural beats. There are countless apps available for Android and IPhone that offer binaural beats for sleep, but I recommend Relax Melodies for IOS and Relax Melodies or Binality for Android.

I have used binaural beats for years and have found there to be many benefits. The most obvious of which is the ability to fall asleep or induce a change in consciousness without the use of drugs or medication. With prescription sleeping pill use on the rise, any effective solution that can induce sleep without chemicals should be explored. Commonly prescribed sleeping pills like Ambien® (Zolpidem) are known to have strange and often terrifying side effects like sleepwalking and sleep eating. Clearly, binaural beats are a better option.

Supplements and Sleep Aids

There are several supplements that can contribute towards a better night sleep. The most important of which is magnesium. Having proper levels of magnesium will not only improve your sleep, but lower your stress, as well. Shawn Stevenson explains:

"Magnesium is a bonafide anti-stress mineral. It helps to balance blood sugar, optimize circulation and blood pressure, relax tense muscles, reduce pain, and calm the nervous system. Yet, because it has so many functions, it tends to get depleted from our bodies rather fast. Magnesium deficiency is likely the number one mineral deficiency in our world today. Estimates show that upwards of 80 percent of the population in the United States is deficient in magnesium. And, some experts say that these numbers are actually conservative. Chances are, you're not getting enough magnesium into your system, and getting your magnesium levels up can almost instantly reduce your body's stress load and improve the quality of your sleep."

You can increase your magnesium levels in several ways. The first way is through direct supplementation, but not all magnesium supplements are created equal. You want to make sure you are taking the right form. Look for magnesium aspartate, malate, glycinate, threonate, or orotate. These forms have higher absorption rates and are more effective. Take 400-800mg of magnesium daily.

Transdermal magnesium supplements are another excellent choice. Magnesium absorbs through the skin incredibly well. Taking a bath with Epsom salts, which are loaded with magnesium, is one option. Another is to apply magnesium skin creams. Look for pharmaceutical grade magnesium chloride hexahydrate skin cream.

A quick word of caution, though. Magnesium supplements should not be taken by anyone with compromised kidney function. They also should not be taken with calcium supplements or dairy, as magnesium can interfere with calcium absorption. Lastly, magnesium supplements can interfere with the effectiveness of other medications, including blood pressure medications, so make sure to speak with your doctor first.

There are also several other natural herbal sleep aids that are worth mentioning. Chamomile tea is an extremely effective and popular herbal sleep aid. It can safely induce sleep, is healthy for you, and is not addictive. Valerian root is another powerful herbal sleep aid that can help you fall asleep when chamomile tea isn't strong enough. Valerian root supplements can be found in most nutrition stores as well as most convenience stores. Keep in mind, however, that Valerian root can cause an adverse reaction when combined with benzodiazepines, such as Xanax® (Alprazolam), Valium® (Diazepam), and Ativan® (Lorazepam), which are commonly prescribed for treating vertigo.

It is also worth pointing out that melatonin can be taken as a sleep aid, as well. I would, however, exercise caution and use this as a short-term solution only. Melatonin is a hormone, and should be treated as such. If used occasionally, it can work fantastically well as a sleep aid. It can also help avoid jet lag by resetting your circadian rhythm when you travel across time zones. If you take a melatonin supplement at the normal bedtime of your new time zone, you will often find that you are not jet lagged the next morning. It should not, however, be used as a long-term solution.

Sleep Tracking

It is a good idea to keep track of your sleep in your journal. It will help you identify the amount of sleep you need to feel your best. Everyone has a different chemical makeup and there is no magic number of hours of sleep required for everyone. The best approach is to keep a log of your sleep and pay close attention to how you feel. In doing this, you will most likely also find a strong connection between your symptoms and the amount of sleep you're getting. If you are getting too little, you will probably find your symptoms getting worse, regardless of your other efforts. If, however, you are getting plenty of high-quality sleep on a nightly basis, you will probably start noticing progress and a reduction in the severity of your symptoms. At the very least, write down the time that you went to sleep and the time you woke up in your journal.

If you keep a basic log, it will be enough information to help you start making connections between your sleep and your symptoms. But you can automate the process and get more detailed information by using a sleep tracker. Over the last several years, there has been an explosion of fitness and sleep tracking products released on the market. I highly recommend purchasing one that tracks your sleep.

Most of the sleep tracking products automatically sense when you fall asleep and wake up, and store all of the data for you. I personally wear the Peak fitness watch from Basis. It tracks my heart rate, sleep cycles, the number of times I toss and turn each night, and the number of times I wake up, even momentarily throughout the night. It tracks my sleep at a deep level that is certainly not necessary for everyone, but, for me, it's extremely helpful data to have.

A less expensive option is offered by a company called Misfit (Misfit.com). Misfit offers wearable fitness and sleep tracking bands for as little as $50 that don't need to be recharged. Instead, the bands use button cell watch batteries to provide six months of uninterrupted use. The Misfit products are just one option. As time goes on, there will be far more advanced sleep and fitness tracking products to choose from.

Conclusion

Sleep is the glue that holds all of your treatment efforts together. It has the power to turbocharge your success or sabotage your recovery. It's hard to imagine that just getting better sleep could be such a powerful tool against your Meniere's disease symptoms. But it's usually the little things, the obvious things that we tend to overlook first. We are programmed from an early age to believe that the answers come in the shape of a pill. While Western medicine and big pharma do an unquestionable amount of good in this world, and at times for this disease, getting back to the fundamentals of health is always a good idea. It builds a foundation for you to springboard to greater and greater heights. The importance of sleep in your treatment and recovery cannot be overlooked.

EXERCISE

"I have always believed that exercise is the key not only to physical health but to peace of mind." – Nelson Mandela

In today's digitally connected world, people seem to live more sedentary lifestyles than ever before. I'm no exception to this. For most of my life, I sat glued to my couch with the best of them. As our technology evolves and makes our lives easier, our need to actually get up and move around has been drastically reduced.

This is by no means a bad thing. Food can now be delivered to us from a few clicks on our smartphones. Live in a big city and need something from the store several blocks away? For a few dollars, an Uber driver will pick you up and drop you off in minutes. These technologies have made our lives easier but come at a cost. Human beings did not evolve to sit in a chair, in a cubicle, facing a computer screen for 8 hours a day. The lazy nature of our modern existence has led to a rise in major health problems for large swaths of the population. Obesity, heart disease, stroke, and diabetes are reaching new heights, never before observed in the population.

Exercise, however, is a powerful and simple tool to fight for your health. But when facing an illness like Meniere's disease, exercise can also be a terrifying prospect. If your symptoms are bad, the thought of even getting out of bed can be overwhelming.

But if you can add exercise into your routine, even the smallest amount, you will experience great benefits in your recovery. Adopting an exercise practice will improve all other aspects of your physical health and, as a consequence, will strengthen your ability to overcome Meniere's disease. It will reduce your stress, improve the quality and quantity of your sleep, and help to build momentum in your treatment. Additionally, it will help to improve and retrain your balance. As you undoubtedly are aware, Meniere's disease can cripple your equilibrium, even when you are not having vertigo attacks. Through exercise, you will find that your balance will slowly improve over time.

In this chapter, I will explore several approaches to exercise as well as best practices to ensure that you are successful. Even if your symptoms are flaring up, staying in bed for days on end is never the right answer. You may not be able to hit the gym and start lifting weights, but you still have options. Understanding those options and the importance of getting yourself up and moving is crucial. Like sleep, we often overlook exercise as a critical component of health, but again, it's usually the simple things that provide the most benefits.

Start Slow By Walking

Exercise does not have to be intense to provide benefit to your treatment and health. In fact, to the contrary, if you are not physically ready for intense exercise, it can be a detriment. The best strategy when starting out is to start slowly. Take your time and build up to a more complete exercise routine.

One of my favorite ways to exercise is to simply go for walks. If you are still having issues with vertigo, walking slowly on a treadmill while holding on to the handrails is a good strategy. The handrails are there to support you and will help you maintain your balance as you walk. Another good option is to use a walking stick or a cane. Even if you don't end up needing it, it's a good idea to keep one with you and will give you an added boost of confidence. Walking with a friend is also a good idea if you are still having frequent vertigo.

If your symptoms are under control, walking outside can be much more entertaining and enjoyable. There's nothing quite like going for a nice walk around a beautiful or interesting place. I prefer to do this without headphones, letting myself get lost in thought. It's like meditation for me. I will turn my cellphone off and walk around for 20-40 minutes, just taking it all in.

When I walk like this, I find I often have insights and ideas into problems I've been working on or facing. There's something about walking that just seems to stimulate the mind. Walking helps decrease my brain fog, as well.

One of my favorite places is a local park called Morakami Gardens. It's a Japanese garden built smack dab in the middle of South Florida with a one-mile walking path. It is one of the most peaceful and beautiful places I have ever been. In fact, it's the spot Megan and I chose to get married. If you can find a place like this near you, it will make your walks far more enjoyable.

Walking is also all that's needed for your body to start releasing endorphins. When you exercise, your brain releases endorphins, your body's "feel good" chemicals. Ever hear someone refer to a runner's high? They're talking about endorphins. The release of endorphins causes your stress levels to go down and your overall feeling of satisfaction to go up. If you are feeling depressed, the endorphins released during exercise will help considerably toward feeling better.

When you feel well enough, find a way to add walking into your daily routine. It is the easiest way to build an exercise practice into your daily life. As your symptoms and health improve, you can build upon this and start adding intensity and complexity, but it's not necessary, especially early on. When starting out, your goal should just be to get yourself up and moving, for a short period of time, every day. It will help build momentum towards greater and greater effort. It will give you the small wins necessary to build motivation and keep you moving forward in your treatment.

Yoga

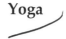

Yoga is another fantastic way to add exercise into your daily routine with benefits that target many of the symptoms of Meniere's disease directly. Yoga combines elements of exercise, meditation, breath control, stretching, and balance. By practicing yoga, you can begin to retrain your equilibrium and improve your sense of balance. Additionally, the meditative aspect of yoga helps to reduce stress while the practice of breath control can help you improve your emotional stability and sense of calm in the face of adversity. All of these elements can help you manage your symptoms.

More importantly, yoga can be a great workout. There are different styles and types of yoga, many of which provide a rigorous workout. You can really get a good sweat going while releasing a strong rush of endorphins. If you are still experiencing a lot of vertigo or dizziness, there are even styles of yoga that are done sitting in a chair. As your symptoms improve, you can easily transition to a more traditional yoga practice.

If you are interested in trying yoga, there are several

good ways to get started. The first is to find a local yoga studio and take a beginners class. There are many different types of yoga, and I recommend trying several different styles to find what resonates with you the most. Yogafinder.com is a good resource to search for yoga studios near you. Otherwise, a simple Google search should also provide a good list of options nearby.

If you don't want to go to a class, you still have options. There are thousands of yoga videos that you can follow along with in the comfort of your home. Amazon.com is a great resource for this. Through Amazon Instant Video, you can stream many different yoga routines, either by renting the titles or purchasing them. For most of the titles, DVDs are available, as well, for easy home viewing on your TV. One of my favorites available on Amazon is a video called "Jing Yoga" that combines elements of yoga and qigong. It's about 75 minutes long and is an excellent routine for beginners and experts alike. YouTube.com is another good resource for yoga routines. A simple search for "Yoga" brings up nearly 6 million results. With YouTube, all the yoga videos are free, and many are only 20-30 minutes in length, which is perfect for beginners.

The only equipment you need to do yoga is a yoga mat, and you can purchase one at most sporting goods stores. You can find them online, as well. I personally prefer the mats that are thicker and provide extra cushioning for your ankles and joints. There is no need to purchase yoga clothes to do yoga. Wearing comfortable exercise clothes is perfectly fine.

In many ways, yoga is the ideal exercise for someone suffering from Meniere's disease. It's definitely worth giving it a try. It has always helped me to improve my balance and reduce my stress.

Cardio

Once I was able to increase the intensity of my exercise, I found that a good cardiovascular workout helped to manage my Meniere's symptoms. A word of caution, though: if you are still experiencing vertigo or dizziness on a regular basis, cardio workouts may not be your best option just yet. When your balance is severely impaired, an intense cardio workout can be outright dangerous. But if you are having some success in managing your symptoms, cardio workouts are a great way to improve your symptoms and get in shape.

I recommend starting out on a treadmill, elliptical, or stationary bike. This way, if you have any difficulties, you have handrails to hold on to. I also recommend starting out slow. Always give yourself a warm-up period of 5 to 10 minutes before you work your way up to higher intensity. You can hurt yourself if you try to go too fast or turn up the resistance too quickly.

Increase the level of difficulty slowly, and over time, for the best results. Your body will thank you for it.

I have always found that cardio workouts not only lower my stress levels, but improve my mood, my energy levels, and my mental clarity, as well. Intense exercise can also radically reduce brain fog and help you to get better sleep.

Once you have a comfortable routine on the stationary equipment, taking your workout outside can make it much more enjoyable. Going for a run or jog through a park or a big city can add an element of novelty to your experience. The sunlight and fresh air can keep you happy and motivated in a way that isn't generally found at the gym. Going for a bike ride outdoors is always a lot of fun, as well, especially if you have company. Exercising with other people helps keep your spirits up. Aim for 20-40 minutes of cardio for maximum benefit.

High-Intensity Interval Training (HIIT)

Once you are comfortable with basic cardio exercise, you can increase your results by incorporating high-intensity interval training into your workout routine. It allows you to reduce the total time of your workouts while increasing the benefits. High-intensity interval workouts have been shown to burn more body fat than traditional cardio workouts and have the added benefit of increasing your metabolism for a period of time after you exercise.

When I was first diagnosed with Meniere's disease, I was not very physically healthy. So once I had the worst of my symptoms under control, I knew I needed to lose weight and get in shape. High-intensity interval training on the elliptical is what ended up working for me. Over a period of about nine months, I was able to lose close to 60 pounds. I would go to the gym at the same time every morning and do about 15 – 20 minutes of HIIT.

The basic principal of high-intensity interval training is to complete a short burst of high-intensity exercise followed by a short resting period of low-intensity exercise. Together, this makes up one interval, which is repeated several more times. HIIT workouts can be done with traditional cardio exercises as well as with weight training and body weight training, though I recommend cardio.

When starting out, try HIIT on the treadmill, elliptical, or stationary bike. Always warm up for 5 to 10 minutes first to prevent injury. There are several different protocols that vary the amount of time spent on the work and rest period of each interval. When first starting out, try 30 seconds of intense exercise with the resistance or speed turned up to a setting that challenges you, followed immediately by a 90-second period at a slower resting pace. During the 90-second rest period, focus on your breathing. Take slow, deep, steady breaths to bring your heart rate back down. Repeat this for a total of four to six, 2-minute intervals, and end with a 5-minute cool down period of low-intensity exercise. As you improve, you can change the ratio of work to rest. Typically, I will do 60 seconds of intense exercise followed by 60 seconds at a resting pace. You can also try 1-minute intervals with 30 seconds of work and 30 seconds of rest.

I find high-intensity interval training to be a powerful practice for getting your body into shape. The more physically healthy you are, the better your body will be able to fight off your Meniere's symptoms. Your body's limited resources will not be stuck dealing with other health and weight related issues. A high-intensity interval training practice is not necessary to get the treatment benefits of exercise, but if you are physically capable, it's a great shortcut to quickly get your body into shape.

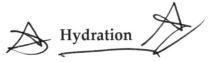

Hydration

No matter what type of exercise you ultimately choose to do, staying well hydrated is incredibly important. Even for a healthy adult, dehydration can cause major problems like dizziness, nausea, cognitive impairment, and much more. Sound familiar? It should. For someone with Meniere's disease, dehydration can put a halt on your progress. You already have enough things to worry about. It's easy to stay hydrated, but it's also easy to forget. Make sure to drink plenty of water and stay well hydrated throughout your whole day, especially when you exercise.

The American Council on Exercise suggests the following guidelines for exercise and hydration:

- "Drink 17-20 ounces of water two to three hours before the start of exercise.
- Drink 8 ounces of fluid 20 to 30 minutes prior to exercise or during warm-up.
- Drink 7-10 ounces of fluid every 10 to 20 minutes during exercise.
- Drink 8 ounces of fluid within 30 minutes after exercising."

A simple way to make sure you are staying well hydrated is to check the color of your urine. The closer it is to colorless, the better hydrated you are. Dark yellow urine is a sign of dehydration.

Journaling and Exercise

Most of my advice on journaling so far has focused on keeping track of specific aspects of your lifestyle to identify the triggers of your symptoms. This is an incredibly valuable practice. It is, however, also very helpful to identify the things that make you feel amazing and improve your symptoms. Discovering your own personal "wellness triggers" is just as important as discovering your Meniere's symptom triggers.

I highly recommend keeping a log of your exercise in your journal. As you experiment and try different types of exercise, keep track of as much information as you can. For example, keep track of when you like to exercise. Some people have better results working out in the morning while others do better in the afternoon. Keep track of the intensity level and duration of your workouts, as well. At a minimum, this will give you a record of your progress. It will also help you identify the level of intensity that benefits you the most.

Keep in mind that it's easy to overdo it if you're not careful. If you push yourself too far past your current abilities, it is entirely possible to experience a setback in your treatment progress. The physical stress of overtraining can increase your symptoms, not to mention, cause injury. Keeping a detailed record of your workouts will help you avoid this outcome or, at the very least, prevent it from happening twice.

You should also keep track of the specific nature of your workouts. If you just completed a HIIT workout on the stationary bike, with 2-minute intervals, 1 minute of work and 1 minute of rest, write it all down. You never know what piece of information might spark a connection in your mind upon review. Write it all down on paper. It will help you find the patterns.

The journaling process can be somewhat automated by wearing a fitness tracker. In the chapter on sleep, I explored these devices and their capacity to track the quantity and quality of your sleep. With exercise, they are a valuable tool for keeping track of your fitness level over time.

The only drawback is that many of these devices cannot distinguish between different types of exercise. Over time, as the technology evolves, I am sure this problem will be addressed. But currently, many of the most common wearable fitness trackers such as the Fitbit, Nike Fuel Band, and the Misfit Shine (that I recommended previously) only track steps taken and an approximation of calories burned.

Unquestionably, this is valuable information to have, and seeing your trends over time can provide helpful insights. But it's a good idea to keep track of more than just steps and calories, at least early on while you are still in the process of learning how your body responds to Meniere's disease. Make it a habit to keep track of the specific details of your workouts.

Setting Goals

When building a new routine, having momentum can really help to make new habits stick. A good way to build momentum with exercise is to set specific goals. The goals you set will depend on many factors: the severity of your symptoms, your current level of fitness, strength and endurance, as well as your previous experience with exercise. The best advice I can give when it comes to setting goals is to make them as short term and obtainable as possible.

There is a specific psychological advantage to this. It boils down to enabling yourself to achieve a large number of continuous small wins. In my experience, succeeding in achieving a goal, no matter how small, provides the motivation and momentum to keep moving forward towards your next goal. For example, if you are just starting or your symptoms are not well-controlled, a small obtainable goal could be to simply walk around your house or neighborhood for five to ten minutes. Successfully completing a 5-minute walk around your house, especially when you didn't think you could, will cause a powerful shift in your mindset. It will also motivate you to do it again. Your progress will build on itself until, one day, you'll find you are able to do things that once seemed impossible.

It's also important to remember that the goals you set do not have to continuously increase the intensity and duration of your workouts. Often, goals of consistency will be more obtainable and more rewarding. It is shockingly easy to convince yourself not to workout. I say this with vast personal experience.

There will always be tough days where you feel unmotivated or tired, regardless of your symptoms. Setting goals to get exercise on a consistent basis is a good way to overcome this. Each small victory will motivate the next, leading to the eventual successful adoption of the habit.

One last thing to consider: it is easier to be consistent with exercise if you work out, to some extent, every day. When it's a part of your daily routine, it's much harder to talk yourself out of it. It becomes just a normal part of your day. By comparison, if you only work out 2 days a week, you may end up having a conversation with yourself about the merits of getting exercise when you are perfectly content to stay on the couch and watch Netflix. Getting exercise, even the smallest amount, every day eliminates the vast majority of these internal debates.

Personal Training

I know it's expensive, but having a personal trainer can be a huge benefit for someone struggling with Meniere's disease. A personal trainer is a one-on-one fitness coach who will metaphorically hold your hand and guide you through the process of getting in shape. They are experts at personal fitness and can teach you the best exercises, proper form, and routines customized specifically for you and your abilities.

For people with balance disorders, this can be really helpful, especially if you are starting out with little to no experience. There are many exercises that can be done safely, from a chair, the floor, or on mats. An experienced personal trainer can help you get into shape regardless of your current limitations or skill level. They can help you set realistic goals and will also design specific workouts and routines.

A good personal trainer also provides several important psychological benefits. The act of committing to a personal trainer and paying for their services gives you the initial motivation to get the ball rolling, and having someone to hold you accountable will keep you motivated once you start. Additionally, a good personal trainer will give plenty of positive reinforcement and encouragement to keep you feeling confident. All of these elements combined create a powerful momentum that will ensure that exercise becomes a habit.

Conclusion

If it seems to be a pattern that some of the most effective strategies for conquering Meniere's disease are the least complicated, you're right. Exercise is no exception. And with a complex idiopathic illness like Meniere's, it's important to take this holistic approach to your health.

Exercise will not be the panacea that many hope for,

but it will help considerably, and it will make all of your other treatment efforts more successful. If you want to get your health back, you have to give yourself every opportunity to heal. Slowly adding exercise into your routine will help to make you healthier as a whole, and consequently will give you the best possible chance of success.

In the next and final section, we will look to the future. Getting your health back and managing your symptoms are both still your first priority, but it is by no means the finish line. Once your symptoms start to improve, it's time to take a different kind of journey – one of personal growth and self-discovery. The great Maya Angelou put it best: "My mission in life is not merely to survive, but to thrive; and to do so with some passion, some compassion, some humor, and some style."

The final section will teach you to define your new limitations accurately, advance your health even further, and to thrive once again.

PART 3:
LEARNING TO
THRIVE

PROGRESS

"Because survival is insufficient."
– Star Trek: Voyager

Now that you've made it this far, let's pause for a moment, take a deep breath, and reflect back on where we've been. Meniere's disease is a terrible illness, with enough conflicting information and reports to make your head spin. So much can go wrong that if you have started to improve simply by chance, you are one of the lucky few. There are so many variables to consider when approaching treatment that it's easy to lose hope. Far too many people do.

But by now, you have learned how to implement a "lifestyle overhaul" to begin getting your symptoms under control. If you have started to have success already, keep it up! You're doing great! If you are still struggling, don't give up. Meniere's disease affects every person differently, and it can take some people more time than others to start seeing results. Even if all of your triggers are outside of your control or understanding, the health benefits of the lifestyle overhaul are profound and will help to manage your symptoms in the long run. Healing takes time. Never give up hope.

So now that you have established new habits and made the necessary lifestyle changes, it's time to learn how to leverage your success to achieve greater progress. You have probably already begun to discover your new limitations. Knowing your physical limits is incredibly important for managing your illness over time.

Once your symptoms are at a more manageable level, you can begin to explore and test the new boundaries of your Meniere's disease by conducting what I like to call lifestyle reversal experiments. During the lifestyle overhaul, you may have had to give up certain things you enjoy, like alcohol and coffee. Now, you can begin to find out if anything can be reintroduced without triggering your symptoms. Giving up coffee was initially a nightmare for me. But by slowly and carefully testing, I was able to discover the amount of coffee (and caffeine) that I could safely consume without triggering my symptoms.

Once you have identified your new boundaries, I will teach you to begin to thrive and experience a level of personal growth that you never dreamed possible. You will learn to reduce brain fog and increase your focus, memory, attention, and productivity. I will teach you about cognitive boosting supplements called Nootropics and states of "peak performance" consciousness called flow states. And finally, you will learn a set of continuing lifestyle management techniques to encourage and nurture your growth and development far into the future.

When you were first diagnosed, you may have felt that a successful, meaningful life of purpose and happiness was impossible. I'm here to tell you that this couldn't be further from the truth. There is always so much hope. No matter where you find yourself, there is always room to improve. Meniere's disease or not, you are capable of incredible things. Never forget that.

Over the years, I have watched in amazement as my life transformed from one that lacked focus and meaning, to one of conviction, clarity, and passionate purpose. When I was first diagnosed, my world crumbled. I was certain that my life was over. You could not have convinced me otherwise. But I eventually made the decision to fight for my health. And once I started seeing results, even the smallest of results, my mindset shifted entirely. I have accomplished more in my 4 years with Meniere's disease than I ever dreamed possible.

Of course, I still have setbacks and bad days. My life is far from perfect. But the overall trajectory is always up. Even if you are never able to get your symptoms fully under control, you can still live your life to the fullest.

LIFESTYLE REVERSAL EXPERIMENTS – FINDING YOUR TRUE LIMITATIONS

"The limits of the possible can only be defined by going beyond them into the impossible."
– Arthur C. Clarke

If you are anything like me, once you have your symptoms under control, you will probably want to start testing what your body can and cannot handle. The strategy so far has been to eliminate all possible and well-known triggers in a sweeping effort to reduce your symptoms. When you are starting out, this is the best way to go. Getting your health back is your top priority.

But once you've made some headway, maintaining every single change you've made can become difficult. One of the things that helped me learn to manage my Meniere's disease in the long term was planning careful experiments to test how specific things affected me. I found that once my symptoms were mostly under control, some of the things I had eliminated from my diet and lifestyle were not, in fact, triggering my symptoms. I've also found that my body reacts differently to certain triggers when I am not actively having symptoms. For example, when my symptoms are acting up, drinking coffee will make me feel worse. But when I'm feeling good, having a cup or two of coffee doesn't trigger me at all.

It has been a long process of learning and discovery for me, but a somewhat enjoyable one. The more I learn about the way my body reacts to Meniere's disease, the more manageable my symptoms become. I can go about my day with greater certainty, knowing how my body will react to my environment. Taking the time to learn and pay attention to your body is worth the effort. It builds confidence and gives you the peace of mind you deserve. Even if you've discovered triggers that are outside of your control, such as environmental allergies or changes in the barometric pressure, understanding how it will affect you will give you more confidence. It will protect you from being blindsided by your symptoms and you will have the opportunity to react ahead of time.

Before I dive in, I want to give you a few words of caution. First of all, understand that if you are comfortable with the lifestyle limitations you have placed on yourself and you are having success in managing your symptoms, you absolutely don't need to test anything. You can skip right on ahead to the next chapter. This step, though empowering, is not necessary. If, however, you are excited to start testing right away, I strongly recommend that you take your time with the following experiments. Start small and work your way up. Don't let your excitement get the best of you. You will be much better off if you go slowly. Patience is your friend here.

Conducting the Reversal Experiments

Before you begin, it's important to think back on all the dietary and lifestyle changes you've made so far. Read back through your journal or any notes you have taken and create a list of everything you have changed. From a diet perspective alone, you have most likely eliminated caffeine, alcohol, and any other food sensitivities you may have discovered. You have restricted your sodium intake and your sugar intake, as well. Hopefully by now, you have been able to identify at least some of your triggers.

Once you have a list of all of your changes, think about what each one means to you. Which changes were the hardest on you? Would you like to be able to have coffee again? Or maybe you would like to be able to drink alcohol with your friends and colleagues. Maybe all of the changes you have had to make upset you and you just want to know the bottom line of what you can and cannot do. All of these thoughts and feelings are perfectly normal. Fortunately, you can go back and test anything you have changed to see how it affects you.

The catch, however, is that you should only test one thing at a time. There is no other way to get to the truth. Meniere's disease is a complex illness and affects everyone differently. If you want to test your new limitations accurately, everything else has to remain perfectly constant. Make sure your routine will stay fixed, as well as your environment and stress levels. This is absolutely necessary.

So now that you understand the requirements, I'll walk you through an example to show you how to carefully test the reintroduction of something you have eliminated.

For me, the thing I missed the most was coffee. I was never a big caffeine drinker to begin with, but I love a good cup of coffee. After my diagnosis, I eliminated caffeine immediately. It was a hard transition to make. The fatigue I was experiencing was already enough to make each day a struggle. Eliminating caffeine made it that much worse. After a few weeks, though, my symptoms started to ease. The pressure in my ears started to lessen. The ringing got quieter. The dizziness started to fade. Once my symptoms were stable, I decided to see if I could handle caffeine again.

I started with a single mug of green tea. Tea generally has less caffeine than coffee. Green tea also has L-theanine, a calming amino acid that I thought would help. Much to my surprise, it didn't trigger my symptoms! I hadn't had any coffee yet, but I felt so optimistic. I continued to drink one cup of green tea each morning until I knew for sure that I could tolerate the caffeine.

After several successful mornings drinking tea, I cautiously drank a half cup of coffee. Once again, I was surprised to find that I felt good. I was thrilled. I slowly and methodically increased the amount caffeine every couple days. Eventually, I discovered that one cup of coffee is perfectly fine, two cups is usually okay, but any more than that and I risk triggering my symptoms. Having this level of understanding is incredibly empowering. By knowing your limitations as specifically as possible, you are able to take back control.

This process is not limited to dietary changes either. You have made many lifestyle changes, as well. You can use the same process to identify the extent that you are affected by environmental triggers. Anything that triggers your symptoms can be carefully tested to discover your actual limitations.

Setting Up the Experiments and Journaling

I strongly recommend keeping detailed notes for any reintroduction experiments you decide to do. Remember, the goal of these tests is to find your true limitations and boundaries. When exploring your triggers, there is always a fine line between what you can handle and what you can't. Keeping a detailed record of how you feel throughout the whole process will help you to identify the line with certainty.

Before you begin testing anything, create a plan. Decide on what you would like to test and write out a schedule to follow. Always stick to your plan, and regardless of what you are testing, start out with small quantities. If you find you aren't triggered immediately, test at that level for several more days to be certain before you start to increase the amount. Make sure to always take your time. If you increase the amount too quickly, you may end up triggering your symptoms without learning anything of value.

As an example, let's say you want to test the reintroduction of wine. A good way to test would be to start out with half a glass. Carefully observe how you react. Take notes in your journal. How do you feel? Are any of your symptoms acting up? No matter how you feel, do not increase the amount until you have tested at this level several more times. Once you know for sure that you can handle half a glass of wine without triggering your symptoms, increase the amount to one full glass. Again carefully observe how your body reacts.

Repeat this process until you either start noticing symptoms or are satisfied with the current amount. If you do start to notice any symptoms, you have already crossed the line. You may find that one to two glasses are fine, but four drinks trigger your symptoms. In this instance, I would consider three drinks to be the line and wouldn't recommend consuming more than one to two on any given occasion. Also, remember that for most people, moderation is important. Even if you are able to tolerate several glasses of wine, that doesn't mean you should indulge every day. It's valuable to know your limitations, but that doesn't mean you should overdo it. You may find that you can have a glass of wine or two every now and then, but more frequent use triggers your symptoms.

If you find that something triggers your symptoms, even in the smallest amounts, having detailed notes will be helpful for you if you decide to retest at some point in the future. Being able to look back and see how something previously affected you will help you to see if your body has adapted or changed at all. Over time, some of my limitations have expanded while others have gotten worse. I can now safely drink coffee, but I can't safely eat ice cream. My allergies, milk, in this case, are a much bigger trigger for me today than they were early on in my diagnosis.

Failures and Frustration

Testing and finding your true limitations can be intensely liberating. The more intimately I understand my illness, the more power I have over my circumstances. Despite this, it has not been an easy road. Many of my early attempts at reintroduction failed. My tests with sodium were the most disappointing.

There's little that I love more than a great meal. I definitely consider myself a foodie. Having to suddenly switch to a low sodium diet was really hard for me, at least for a while. The improvement in my symptoms made it worthwhile, but I desperately hoped I would be able to enjoy food again without constantly worrying about sodium content.

Long story short, years later, I'm still worried about sodium content. I've tested and retested it over the years, and to this day consuming too much sodium is still my biggest trigger. This kind of let down is never fun. As you start testing, you will undoubtedly run into the same frustrations. I know how hard it can be, especially if you find that you can't tolerate something at all, something you never wanted to give up in the first place.

If you find yourself facing failure with these tests, the best advice I can give you is to try to reframe your perspective. We have to make the most of the life we've been given. Sometimes, that means making tradeoffs. But ultimately, what's more important than our health and well-being? Give it enough time and you will adapt. It may be hard initially, but I promise you'll get used to any changes you end up having to make permanently.

It only took a couple of weeks to find that I was actually okay with the low sodium diet. I found myself noticing the flavors of the actual ingredients and the food itself. And as time went on, I learned more about the sodium content in most common foods. Eventually, it became almost like an intuitive sense. I still read nutrition labels, but if I'm not able to, I can keep myself out of trouble with my instincts and general understanding. At this point, the low sodium diet is just a part of my life. At times, it's an inconvenience, but it's nothing I can't handle.

Also, it's important to point out that as time passes, your body will change. Just because you can't tolerate something now doesn't mean you won't ever be able to tolerate it. I have a lot more leeway with my lifestyle today than I used to. I find that despite the fact that sodium still triggers me, I don't have to be as strict with my diet as I was four years ago. I don't actively try to overdo it with salt, but if I do, I'm usually okay and have time to make adjustments before my symptoms are triggered. Always remember that it's perfectly fine to go back and retest in the future.

Warning Signs

When you are conducting the reintroduction experiments, it's important to understand that your symptoms won't always be triggered immediately. It's completely possible to feel fine on the day of the test only to wake up the next morning with symptoms. This also applies to your daily life. If your health has been stable and your symptoms are under control, you most likely won't get vertigo right away. It's usually much more subtle than that, and learning to identify the warning signs is critical.

For me, the warning signs follow a specific progression. If I eat too much sodium at dinner, I will immediately get brain fog. This usually carries over to the next morning. Brain fog is always my first warning sign. If I were to keep eating a high sodium diet, the brain fog would intensify until one morning I would wake up with ear pressure and much louder ringing in my ears. I would start experiencing a general feeling of dizziness next – not vertigo, but a constant low-level dizziness – until finally, I would end up having a vertigo attack.

I have had plenty of brain fog, ear pressure, and dizziness, but I have not had a vertigo attack in several years now. Anytime I start to notice any of the warning signs, I immediately start another temporary "lifestyle overhaul" until the symptoms diminish. Everyone experiences Meniere's disease differently, but if you start to notice warnings signs, I suggest doing the same. The longer you wait, the longer it will take for your symptoms to return to a more manageable level. Identifying your early warning signs will help you avoid this.

It's a Process

It can be helpful to view your treatment as a continual process of self-discovery. You experienced a major change in your biology and, slowly, you are getting to meet your new self. At times, you may be surprised to find you have a hidden strength and resolve that you never knew. You are much stronger than you think.

The lifestyle reversal experiments are no exception. It's a continuous process of growth and learning. You will find your boundaries and understand them better with time and experimentation. It won't happen all at once, and it definitely won't happen easily. But with a little bit of patience and elbow grease, you will discover your true limitations and feel a new sense of freedom.

GROWTH

"Don't ask yourself what the world needs.
Ask yourself what makes you come alive and
then go do that. Because what the world needs
is people who have come alive."
– Howard Thurman

Starting right now, I am going to teach you how to thrive. Getting a handle on your symptoms and learning to live with Meniere's disease is just the beginning. The rest of this book will be an exploration of strategies for significantly increasing your quality of life. No matter what stage you are at in the treatment process, you can begin to seek a life of happiness and meaningful purpose. You can start to grow and improve.

Even if you are still limited, you can learn how to live a fulfilling life. Martin Luther King Jr. once said, "If I cannot do great things, I can do small things in a great way." I love this idea; it's so freeing. Even if you cannot achieve exactly what you had originally intended, you can still find your place in the world and make a meaningful impact.

I have found that by consciously living a purposeful

life, my world has expanded greatly. Everyone has something special to share with the world; you just have to look within yourself and discover what it is.

Finding the Opportunity within Adversity

The universe has a twisted sense of humor.

Sometimes, the forces of nature seem to conspire against us like we are unwitting participants in some kind of cosmic reality show that needs more drama. For whatever reason, life maintains the perverse habit of throwing us curve balls when we least expect it. Throughout our lives, we all experience heartbreak, pain, tragedy, and hardship in all colors, shapes, and sizes.

But every once in a while, we open our eyes to find our world has suddenly turned itself upside down and shattered into pieces. In an instant, everything can change. The rug is ripped out from under us faster than we can blink, taking our sense of purpose with it. The feeling of loss can overwhelm you.

Facing this sudden new reality, violently forced upon your ego, you find yourself standing at a precipice. The weight of your new circumstances can crush you if you let it. But if you can bravely recognize this moment for what it truly is, a new path will emerge. Adversity offers us the rare opportunity for personal growth and self-actualization. A diagnosis of

Meniere's disease is no exception.

Often, after the initial shock wears off, we start to realize what truly matters: that life is short, and we only get one go at it.

So many of us stay blindly caught up in the rat race of life and never take the time to enjoy it or even appreciate what we have until its gone. We feel invincible until that unfortunate moment when the universe shows us otherwise.

In a beautiful irony, however, clarity can be found within the chaos. A new, stronger sense of purpose can rise from the ashes of a torched worldview.

After surviving a near-death experience, Adam Braun, author of *The Promise of a Pencil* and founder of the inspiring nonprofit Pencils for Promise, writes, "But I was also forever altered because I now knew that my life had purpose. Out of catastrophe emerged clarity. When faced with the prospect of death, something deep within me fought back. I was here for a reason."

No matter how bad things may seem, now or in the future, there will always be the possibility of happiness, success, and a meaningful life of purpose. You just have to know where to look to find it.

We only get one shot at this crazy game of life. The real question is, how can you make the most of the hand you've been dealt? Finding a new sense of purpose is crucial, and passion is the key.

The first step is to remain calm and begin to identify

your options. You need to gain an understanding of what is still within your control, and discover what choices there are to make.

In his book *The Obstacle is the Way*, Ryan Holiday offers a modern take on the Stoic philosophy of finding opportunity within adversity: "There are a few things to keep in mind when faced with a seemingly insurmountable obstacle. We must try: To be objective. To control emotions and keep an even keel. To choose to see the good in a situation. To steady our nerves. To ignore what disturbs or limits others. To place things in perspective. To revert to the present moment. To focus on what can be controlled. This is how you see the opportunity within the obstacle."

The emotional weight of a life-changing adversity like Meniere's disease can make rational thought seem impossible. But if you stay calm and take inventory of your life, you will see that all is not lost. Your life path may have taken a sharp right turn, but change is not inherently good or bad. It's up to you find the meaning.

Ask yourself the following questions:

- What opportunities are still available to me?
- What skills do I have? What are my unique gifts?
- What are some of the common themes of my previous life's work?
- What brings me joy and excitement?
- How can I help or serve others?

You may find yourself cut off from your previous life's work, but that doesn't mean you can't still pursue your interests. You just have to get a little bit creative. Explore your passions from a new angle, with a new approach, and you just might be pleasantly surprised to find yourself happier than you were before.

As much as you are capable, try new things. Discover what lights that fire in your mind. It's okay to not have all the answers; as the famous cliché goes, "It's about the journey, not the destination."

Also, whenever possible, share your gifts with the world. Nothing will give you a greater sense of purpose and satisfaction than effectively serving others. Not everyone will change the world, but it's within all of us to at least make our mark by helping others.

By doing something that you love, that gets you excited and brings you joy, while at the same time serving others, you will likely find success and a clear sense of purpose.

Make no mistake, finding passion and a new sense of purpose in your life will not be easy. It will take courage and strength and a deep sense of resolve. Don't sell yourself short, though. When you are struggling in the face of a seemingly impossible adversity, you may be banged up, bloody, and bruised, but you are still standing.

One my favorite poems, "The Oak Tree" by Johnny Ray Ryder Jr, sums it up the best:

"A mighty wind blew night and day.
It stole the oak tree's leaves away,
Then snapped its boughs and pulled its bark
Until the oak was tired and stark.

But still the oak tree held its ground
While other trees fell all around.
The weary wind gave up and spoke,
How can you still be standing Oak?

The oak tree said, I know that you
Can break each branch of mine in two,
Carry every leaf away,
Shake my limbs, and make me sway.

But I have roots stretched in the earth,
Growing stronger since my birth.
You'll never touch them, for you see,
They are the deepest part of me.

Until today, I wasn't sure
Of just how much I could endure.
But now I've found, with thanks to you,
I'm stronger than I ever knew."

To find success, you will eventually need to step outside of your comfort zone. The problem is, your brain will come up with a million excuses not to: "It's just not the right time yet" or "That would never work." This is fear, plain and simple. Fear of failure, fear of the unknown, fear of shame, fear of uncertainty.

The reality is that everyone who has ever accomplished anything of great value has faced the same fear. You must be brave in the face of this fear and realize it is far better to take a leap of faith and stumble than never to have tried at all. Because behind every adversity lies growth and learning and opportunity. Face the fear knowing that, above all, it's a sign that you are on the right path.

Lifestyle Replacements

While the lifestyle reversal experiments are a good way to discover what you can and cannot handle, it's not your only option. Instead of reintroducing variables you have removed, you can always try to find suitable replacements instead. There are viable alternatives for many of the common dietary triggers of Meniere's symptoms. I'll give you a few interesting examples.

Alcohol

Removing alcohol entirely from your life can be tricky for some people. Not in a physical sense, but because it's so pervasive in our culture. Not everyone is triggered by alcohol, but I want to suggest an interesting alternative, one that's existed for thousands of years in relative obscurity. It's called kava, and it has only become more widespread over the last several decades.

Kava, it turns out, is a nice alternative to alcohol. It's safer, non-addictive, natural, and most importantly, doesn't trigger my Meniere's symptoms. For more than 3,000 years, the South Pacific Islanders have celebrated this special plant. To this day, it remains a cornerstone of their culture, a celebrated aspect of their religious ceremonies, social lives, and politics. To the natives of Vanuatu, Fiji, and many other South Pacific island nations, it has been a cherished tradition for millennia.

Kava is a relaxing tea made with the roots of the kava plant (*Piper Methysticum*), and according to the community at Kavaforums.com, "the effects of kava include:

- Relaxation
- A sense of well-being
- Increase in alertness
- Pain relief
- Muscle Relaxation
- Relief from Insomnia
- Treatment for Generalized Anxiety Disorder (GAD)
- Treatment of Elevated Anxiety Disorder
- Treatment for Depression

- Increase in Sleep Quality

Kava has been demonstrated to be a very effective treatment for anxiety; equal to Buspirone and Opipramol and more effective than valerian or St. John's Wort, without the side effects associated with benzodiazepines such as tolerance and negative cognitive effects and sedation."

If you decide to try kava, make sure to practice moderation. Kava has never triggered my Meniere's symptoms, but everybody's biology is different. Start slowly to make sure it doesn't negatively affect you. Kava has what is known as a reverse tolerance. Unlike alcohol, where the more you drink, the higher your tolerance gets, with kava it's the opposite. The more often you drink it, the less it takes to feel the effects. Because of this, some people may not experience any effects the first several times they drink kava. The active alkaloids in kava, called kavalactones, have to build up in your system first.

Like all natural products, kava has been known to have side effects. It has been reported to cause headaches, nausea, and double vision in some users. Drinking kava too frequently can also dry out your skin, though this is completely reversible. There are no reported cases of death caused by kava overdose.

A word of caution though: years ago, there was a report of liver health problems as a result of kava use that resulted in kava restrictions in several countries, but not in the US. In follow-up studies, however, traditional kava use was found to be safe and most of the kava restrictions have been reversed. Kava has been used in the South Pacific Islands for thousands of years with no evidence of a higher than normal rate of liver problems. That being said, if you have a history of liver problems, you should avoid kava completely.

Kava can have a strong negative reaction when combined with many different prescription and over-the-counter medications, including narcotic pain medications and benzodiazepines, such as Xanax® (Alprazolam), Valium® (Diazepam), and Ativan® (Lorazepam), which are commonly prescribed for vertigo.

SPEAK WITH YOUR DOCTOR FIRST BEFORE TRYING KAVA AND MAKE SURE IT WILL NOT INTERACT WITH ANY OF YOUR MEDICATIONS.

If you do decide to try kava, the best way to consume it is when it's prepared in the traditional way, with water and ground kava root. Instant kava products are a great alternative, as well. Like instant coffee, you just add water and you're ready to go.

You can find a list of several reputable kava vendors at Mindovermenieres.com/bookresources.

Caffeine

↑ in energy

Caffeine is, by far, the most commonly used drug in the world. Between coffee, tea, soda, and energy drinks, it's probably safe to assume that before your Meniere's symptoms appeared, you consumed caffeine in one way or another. If you can no longer tolerate caffeine without triggering your symptoms, there are several replacements to consider trying on days when you need a boost to your energy levels.

First up is Vitamin B12, one of the eight different B vitamins and utilized throughout the body. It plays a role in nervous system function, brain function, and blood cell formation. B12 has long been recognized for its stimulating properties, especially for people who have a B vitamin deficiency. Vitamin B12 also plays a factor in the production of Melatonin, so not only will you get an energy boost during the day, but better sleep at night. There are countless varieties of B12 supplements on the market, but I recommend the sublingual form for faster absorption.

A healthy dose of green vegetables can also boost your energy. If you have ever been to a premium grocery store like Whole Foods, you have probably seen an isle with packets and jars of "superfood" greens powders. These products are dried and powdered blends of nutrient-dense vegetables and grasses. You simply add it to a glass of water, mix it up, and drink it down.

There are numerous companies offering dehydrated greens powders and the results are generally the same. One serving of these powders packs a massive nutrient punch. It's not meant to replace eating vegetables, but it is a fantastic way to load up on micro and macro nutrients that will give you a boost of natural energy.

The next replacement that has worked well for me is called Tyrosine. Tyrosine is an amino acid and is converted by the body into dopamine and norepinephrine. By taking the supplement L-Tyrosine or the more bioavailable (higher absorption rate) N-Acetyl-L-Tyrosine as a supplement, you can get a boost in energy as well as improved mood and focus. It's much more subtle in effect than caffeine, which is a stimulant, but Tyrosine is an extremely common ingredient in energy drinks for a reason. It can give you energy after a rough night of sleep and a cognitive boost, as well.

These three alternatives are just a starting point. There are many foods, ingredients, and supplements that can provide an overall feeling of energy. Always proceed with caution though. Start with small doses and work your way up to avoid possibly triggering your symptoms.

Conquering Brain Fog

When battling Meniere's disease, with all its hardships and difficulties, I find that often it's the lesser symptoms like brain fog that are the most frustrating. Even when you have gained some semblance of control over the vertigo, learned to ignore the tinnitus, and live an overall healthy lifestyle, brain fog can quickly derail any momentum you may have working for you. It can bring your productivity to a grinding halt and can rob you of precious hope.

Brain fog is an insidious phenomenon. It will not handicap you like vertigo, but can impair your quality of life considerably. So what is brain fog? Loosely defined, brain fog is a form of fluctuating cognitive impairment that affects concentration, executive function, decision making, memory, and word recall. For sufferers of Meniere's disease and many other chronic illnesses, brain fog is a seemingly ever-present clouding of consciousness and an unfortunate reality.

Brain fog can drastically reduce your creativity while making it hard to recall words and carry on an effective conversation. Not to mention the fuzzy feeling of fatigue and lack of motivation that many people experience. It's hard to get anything accomplished when your mental energy levels are low and you feel unmotivated. Possibly the most frustrating aspect of brain fog, however, is the way it can affect your memory. Losing focus and attention is one thing, but forgetting your responsibilities and promises are another thing entirely. It has the power to damage your personal relationships.

But fear not, there are powerful ways to fight back against brain fog.

I've found many strategies that are extremely effective. It's worth pointing out, however, that all of the lifestyle changes I suggest in part two of this book will improve brain fog. Eating a healthy diet, meditation, stress reduction, exercise, and getting better sleep will all play a role in reducing brain fog. More importantly, they will provide a foundation to build on and will make everything else I recommend far more effective.

The following methods, however, are much more direct and combat the symptoms of brain fog at the chemical level. There are also techniques for managing the specific symptoms of brain fog.

The following chapters will cover techniques that will not only improve brain fog, but will improve your overall cognitive abilities. The same principals and strategies that will enable you to thrive will drastically reduce, if not eliminate, your brain fog.

Nootropic (Cognitive Enhancing) Supplements

Disclaimer: Remember, I am not a doctor or a medical professional. Everyone is different and all supplements can have side effects. Please speak to your doctor or medical professional before taking any new supplement or drug. The following are my personal opinions only!

Of everything I have found to increase focus, attention, productivity, and reduce brain fog, nothing has worked faster or been more effective for me than Nootropic supplements. Think of Nootropics as performance enhancing substances, but for your brain. Aside from giving you a cognitive boost, many offer the added benefit of being neuroprotective, as well, meaning they protect your brain's neurons from injury and degeneration.

So, what are Nootropics? Any herbs, vitamins, supplements, or medications that are known to improve and enhance cognitive functions such as concentration, attention, and memory are considered to be Nootropic compounds.

Caffeine, for example, is considered a Nootropic substance. But caffeine is a common trigger for Meniere's symptoms and is likely not a good option. If you happen to find that you are not triggered by caffeine, a cup of coffee can help to temporarily decrease brain fog and give you a nice cognitive boost.

There are, however, a wide variety of other compounds, both artificial and natural, that fall under this umbrella. Many have been extensively studied and researched, though some have not been.

Nootropic supplements fall into several different categories that broadly define how they work. Some Nootropics work by affecting the neurotransmitter acetylcholine. Higher acetylcholine levels in the brain are linked to an increase in focus, concentration, and executive function. Some compounds, such as Choline Bitartrate and Alpha GPC, directly increase the production of acetylcholine, while others, such as Huperzine-A, block the breakdown of acetylcholine, leaving more available. Others still, including the "Racetam" family of Nootropics, increase the effectiveness of acetylcholine. Piracetam, one of the oldest and more widely studied Nootropics, has also been shown to reduce the frequency of recurrent vertigo (Ncbi.nlm.nih.gov/pubmed/10338110).

There are several Nootropics that work by increasing the level of the neurotransmitter dopamine. Having an increased level of dopamine can reduce stress, depression, and anxiety. It's also known to enhance motivation, confidence, and focus. Lastly, some Nootropics affect the metabolism and optimize the energy supply of your brain cells. Vinpocetine, for instance, promotes increased blood flow to the brain causing an increase in oxygen and glucose, which form ATP, the energy source for the neurons in your brain.

A lot of the Nootropic supplements tend to work best when combined. These combinations are known as Nootropic stacks and often create a powerful synergistic effect. Though some people create these stacks on their own, many companies offer pre-formulated combinations.

One of the most common Nootropic stacks is the combination of caffeine and L-theanine (a calming amino acid found in green tea). This combination provides the cognitive benefits of the caffeine with the calming effect of the L-theanine for focused concentration without jitteriness.

I have personally tried many pre-formulated products, but the one that I feel comfortable recommending at this time is a product called Alpha Brain, produced by Onnit Labs (Onnit.com/alphabrain/). I have had tremendous success with this product over the last couple of years. Not to mention, Alpha Brain is the only product I know of that has undergone third party double blind placebo controlled clinical testing. The results were highly positive.

I find that on days when my brain fog is at its worst, a single dose of Alpha Brain increases my clarity and ability to pay attention for 4-6 hours. Often it's the difference between having enough focus to get my work done or not. It improves my memory recall and decreases that notorious "tip of the tongue syndrome" where you can't recall words. Alpha Brain has ingredients such as alpha-GPC that increase acetylcholine production while at the same time blocking its breakdown with Huperazine-A, for maximum benefit. It also contains several potent antioxidants as part of the formulation.

Even when I'm not suffering from brain fog, Nootropics like Alpha Brain help me to stay focused and engaged with whatever I'm working on for long periods of time. Keep in mind, though, Nootropics are not miracle drugs. The drug "NZT" from the movie *Limitless* that turned Bradley Cooper into a super genius after just one dose sadly doesn't exist. But Nootropics do help me to stay focused and combat brain fog, and have for a while now. It was a defining moment in my treatment and in my life when I realized that careful supplementation could help to optimize my brain and reduce brain fog.

If you are interested in researching Nootropics further, you can find more information and resources at Mindovermenieres.com/bookresources.

Creativity Exercises

Life constantly requires us to creatively solve problems and come up with ideas, but brain fog can make this extremely difficult. It's hard to come up with good ideas when your brain feels like mush. You can reduce the impact of brain fog and strengthen your creative abilities by adopting a simple creativity practice into your daily routine.

The basic technique here is simple. Every day, grab a piece of paper and a pen, and choose a topic. Next, come up with a list of ten ideas based on that topic. For example, yesterday my list was 10 things I could do to reduce stress. Some other examples for list topics could be: 10 ideas for products I could invent for my cat, 10 gift ideas for my significant other, or 10 things that could help me at work. Coming up with a theme is part of the exercise.

This practice is like lifting weights with your brain. After coming up with 6 or 7 ideas, it usually gets hard, and I tend to break a mental sweat. This is the goal. You are forcing your mind to think hard and generate ideas.

I highly recommend the best-selling book *Becoming an Idea Machine* by Claudia Altucher. It provides 6 months' worth of daily prompts for this practice and is an excellent resource for learning more about this method. You can also find hundreds of idea list prompts at Ideas-a-day.com.

I've practiced this daily for more than a year and have found that I constantly have a flow of ideas when I need them. It has counteracted the creative impairment of brain fog quite well. I have also found that by forcing myself to do this exercise when my brain fog is at its worse, it reduces the severity. Nothing seems to get my brain firing like forced concentration and the "ah ha" moment that precedes a great idea.

I have found this to work with other creative practices, as well. If writing is more your style, set aside time daily to write. You can find hundreds of creative writing prompts at Reddit.com/r/WritingPrompts. I find writing to be a powerful way to reduce brain fog. Once, after suffering a ten-day bout with the flu, my brain fog was the worst it had been in months. I decided to try writing creative fiction for the first time ever by responding to various writing prompts I found online. It didn't get rid of my brain fog completely, but it improved it enough that I could get work done.

If you consider yourself more an artist than a writer, set aside time each day to create or work on your art. The principle is the same. You are taking time every day to strengthen your creative muscles. The more regularly you do this, the less your creativity will be affected when brain fog strikes and the more creative you will be overall.

How to Improve Your Memory

Before I get into specific techniques, I want you to grasp one thing right now: your memory is not a fixed trait. Memory is a skill that can be learned and enhanced through training. This simple truth is cause for hope.

For many people, including myself, brain fog can severely impair your memory and recall ability. The impact, however, can be lessened by understanding the inherent strengths and weaknesses of our memory capabilities and learning techniques to leverage the strengths.

In general, people are bad at remembering numbers, lists of words, and abstract concepts. However, people are usually very good at remembering images, stories, physical locations, and places they know.

The basic technique is to take difficult to remember information and transform it into something that our brains can easily remember. This practice is known as "linking" and all it takes is a little bit of imagination.

Linking Technique

Linking is a powerful memory trick and is easy to start using right away. You simply take the thing you wish to remember and turn it into a story with vivid, exaggerated images in your mind.

To demonstrate, I will walk you through the process of remembering the following ten-item grocery list: **Eggs, Beef, Green Beans, Celery, Fish, Chicken, Guacamole, Bananas, Ice Cream, and Orange Juice.**

Now, read the following ridiculous story slowly and

as you read, **really try to vividly imagine the scene in your mind:**

The Easter Bunny is sitting on top of a ladder in the middle of a field, violently throwing giant, brightly colored **Eggs** at **Cows** grazing in the field. The cows moo loudly in protest. Across the field, Mickey Mouse is laying in a large hammock, made out of a single giant **Green Bean**. Mickey is drinking a bucket-sized Bloody Mary with a whole stalk of **Celery** sticking out. Suddenly, Mickey turns to see a large **Fish** with human legs, chasing a two headed **Chicken** across the nearby road. The two headed chicken dives into an Olympic-sized swimming pool filled with **Guacamole** on the other side of the road to hide from the fish. The fish gives up on the chicken and heads home and, to his delight, finds his bathtub is filled with a massive **Banana** Split **Ice Cream** Sundae. He eats the entire thing and turns on the faucet to clean out the tub only to find heavy pulp **Orange Juice** coming out. He shrugs and takes a drink.

Now, go back and reread the last paragraph several more times, and really imagine it in as much detail as possible. Once you've done that, put the book down and grab a pen and a piece of paper.

In your mind, I want you to play back the story. Mentally walk through the details of the story, and as you get to each image, write down the corresponding grocery item it represents. For instance, when you get to the cows, you write down beef.

I'm willing to bet you were able to remember the whole list. Pretty amazing, right?

By taking the information you need to remember and transforming it into a vivid and imaginative story, you will have a much easier time remembering. When choosing images and scenarios for your story, the more extreme, exaggerated, disgusting, crazy, humorous, and dramatic, the better. We remember things that invoke emotion, whether shock, disgust, laughter, sadness, etc., with much greater clarity than mundane, random facts.

Memory Palace Technique

The memory palace technique builds on the concept of linking. It is fun to use, easy to learn, and has been around since the time of Ancient Rome.

Earlier I mentioned that people are naturally very good at remembering places they know. This is because a large amount of mental energy is devoted to navigating our environment. I'll give you an example:

Close your eyes, and imagine you are standing at the front door of the home that you grew up in. Open the door and mentally walk through the layout of your childhood home. You can probably remember the layout with a surprising level of detail. You may be surprised to find you can remember the layout of most places you visit frequently.

Combining this natural tendency of memory with the vivid imagery of linking creates a powerful framework for remembering information.

By **mentally** placing vivid images that represent what you are trying to remember (linking) throughout a well-known location, you can easily recall the images later on by walking back through the location in your mind. The term "memory palace" refers to any location you can easily visualize and use to store and remember information.

To get started, first choose a location that you know perfectly, such as your current home. Next, identify 10 different locations within your home, in order of how you would walk through your home. For instance, the first location could be your driveway, the second location might be standing outside your front door, the third location, the room on the inside of the front door, and so on. Make sure each hallway or room is counted only once.

Once you have identified 10 distinct locations within your home, close your eyes and mentally walk through the locations, in order, several times. Once you have it firmly in your mind, you can populate each location with an image that corresponds to what you are trying to remember.

If you think back to our grocery list example, you could imagine a giant Easter Bunny carrying a basket of large **Eggs** at the base of your driveway, while a herd of cows rushes towards your front door (representing **Beef**). Inside your front door, you find Mickey Mouse drinking a bucket-sized Bloody Mary with a full stalk of **Celery** sticking out. You get the idea.

When each of the 10 locations has an image stored, you should be able to recall each image by mentally walking through the memory palace. Give it a try! The first time I recalled a list correctly, I felt like I had discovered a super power.

A simple variation of this technique is to use physical places on your body, rather than rooms in a house, as locations to store information. First, you need to remember the following ten locations on your body, in order.

1. The top of your head
2. Your nose
3. Your mouth
4. Your ears
5. Your throat
6. Your shoulders
7. Your collar (by your collar bones)
8. Your fingers
9. Your stomach
10. Your butt

Go through this list several times and touch each location on your body as you read the list. It will help commit it to memory. Once you have it down, you can use each location to store a piece of information. For example, going back again to the grocery list example, you could imagine the Easter bunny sitting on the top of your head, holding a basket of **Eggs**. Next you could imagine a hot dog sticking out of each nostril of your nose to represent **Beef**. Next, picture yourself chomping on a giant, baseball bat-sized stalk of **Celery**, and so on. Once you have an image for each location, you can easily recall it by mentally going through the list of locations on your body.

With all of these techniques, you can learn to do incredible, seemingly impossible things, like memorizing a shuffled deck of cards. To my surprise, I was able to learn to do this with only several hours of practice. There are even international memory competitions where participants compete with each other to accomplish insane feats of memory. The world record for memorizing a shuffled deck of cards is a mind-blowing 21.9 seconds.

Dual-N-Back Training

In recent years, brain researchers have found that by practicing a simple exercise called the N-Back task, you can not only increase your working memory but raise your IQ points and fluid intelligence (the capacity to think logically and solve problems in novel situations), as well. The N-Back task was originally developed as a way to test a person's short-term working memory. But when turned into a game, it can be used as a training tool to improve working memory and fluid intelligence. There are many variations, but a version of the game called Dual-N-Back is the one I recommend.

I won't mince words; it's incredibly difficult and not what I would call fun. At times, it can be incredibly frustrating. But it actually works, and if you keep at it, you will benefit substantially.

The Dual-N-Back game itself is typically played on a computer. You start with what looks like a tic-tac-toe board and watch as a square appears in one of the 8 locations (the middle spot isn't used), while at the same time, a letter of the alphabet is spoken aloud. After a few seconds, the square vanishes and reappears in a new randomized location on the tic-tac-toe board with a new letter being spoken aloud. Each time this happens, you have to identify if either the new location or the new letter (or both) matches the previous location or spoken letter.

Starting out at level 1, it's not that difficult as you only have to remember the position and spoken letter from one move backward. But as you move through the levels, it becomes increasingly more challenging. At level 2, you are comparing the current location and spoken letter to the location and spoken letter from 2 moves back. Then 3 moves back, then 4 moves, and so on. There are times when it feels like it's impossible, but don't give up. It may take a couple days, but your brain will adapt and form the new connections necessary to break through. It's sort of like power lifting with your brain. You'll improve, slowly but surely.

If you can practice for 20 minutes a day for one month, you will be able to achieve a major boost in your working memory and an increase in IQ points. It's tedious work, but the payoff is huge. You can find a free open source version of the Dual-N-Back game at Mindovermenieres.com/bookresources.

Flow States

One of the most exciting things I've come across in the last couple of years is the research into the consciousness state of peak performance, more commonly known as the flow state. I was delighted to find that the rare and incredible feeling of "being in the zone" that I have experienced from time to time throughout my life, actually had a name. But more importantly, discovering how to have these flow state experiences more often has had a profoundly positive effect on my Meniere's disease. So let me back up for a second and define a couple of things.

First off, it will be helpful to understand what a flow state is. The term "flow state" was originally coined by psychologist Mihaly Csikszentmihalyi in his groundbreaking book, *Flow: The Psychology of Optimal Experience*. Csikszentmihalyi's research set out to discover the fundamental underpinnings of happiness and creativity in the human experience. He was intensely fascinated by artists who became so lost in their work that they would forgo food, water, and sleep. Throughout his research, he discovered that many people, from all walks of life, often reported a similar set of experiences and described them as being some of the happiest and most fulfilling moments of their lives. In interviews, Csikszentmihalyi describes the flow state as "being completely involved in an activity for its own sake. The ego falls away. Time flies. Every action, movement, and thought follows inevitably from the previous one, like playing jazz. Your whole being is involved, and you're using your skills to the utmost."

Many people have experienced this, or something similar, at some point in their lives. When you find yourself so in the zone that time seems to slow down or speed up. Your ability to focus becomes intensely amplified. Your senses become heightened, and you become totally immersed in the present moment. Your brain feels as though it has been supercharged. Sometimes it's as simple as getting lost in conversation with an interesting person, or being so absorbed in a book that hours passed in what felt like minutes. Other times, it can feel almost transcendental or even mystical in nature. I didn't know these experiences were replicable. I was intrigued.

The Science of Flow

In his best-selling book *The Rise of Superman*, Steven Kotler explains that during flow states, our brain releases a potent neurochemical cocktail of dopamine, serotonin, norepinephrine, endorphins, and anandamide. All of these are strong performance-enhancing chemicals.

For a long time, scientists believed that during a flow experience, the prefrontal cortex of the brain is more active than usual. Given the massive boost in performance found in the flow state, this would make sense as the prefrontal cortex is the area of the brain responsible for high level cognitive function. But amazingly, the opposite is true. "'We had it backward,' he says. 'In flow, parts of the PFC [Prefrontal Cortex] aren't becoming hyperactive; parts of it are temporarily deactivating. It's an efficiency exchange. We're trading energy usually used for higher cognitive functions for heightened attention and awareness.'"

Steven Kotler's organization The Flow Genome Project has been researching flow states for years, and identifying what happens in the brain during flow was only the beginning. They also discovered replicable flow state triggers, conditions that increase the number of instances of flow in a person's life. I will cover these in detail, but first, it's important to understand the connection between flow and chronic illness.

Flow and Chronic Illness

On an episode of author Dave Asprey's podcast Bulletproof Radio (Episode 109), Steven Kotler described his struggle with Lyme disease which left him crippled for years, and how he used flow states to bring himself back from the brink. It's an incredible story and relates somewhat closely to my experience with flow's effect on Meniere's disease. Steven was out of options and his doctors were stumped. The following is an excerpt from the podcast transcript:

> I was going to kill myself because all I was going to be from that point on was a burden to my friends and my family. I was not a functioning human being at all. I was lucid for half an hour a day. At the worst point of it, a friend of mine shows up at the front door and says, "We're going surfing." I looked at him, I was like, "You're out of your mind we're going surfing. I can't walk across the room. I can't make it to my kitchen." "We're going surfing."
>
> She wouldn't shut up and wouldn't leave. Finally I was like, "You know what? I don't care. We'll go surfing today. What is the worst that could happen?" They literally had to walk

me to the car. They put me into the car. This was in LA. We went to a place called Sunset Beach which is really like the wimpiest beginner wave in the entire world. It was summer so the waves were even smaller.

The tide was really low. It was a crap day. The waves were two feet high. They gave me a board the size of a Cadillac. The bigger the board, the easier it is to catch a wave. They literally had to walk me out to the break. People had to hold my arms and kind of carry me out to the break.

I got out there. I was at it for about 30 seconds when the wave came. It had been a really long time since I had surfed at that point. Muscle memory seemed to take over. I spun my board, paddled, and I popped up. I popped up into an entirely new dimension. I'm standing on my board and I've got near panoramic vision. Time has slowed down and most importantly, I feel great. I feel better than I've felt in three years. My muscles don't hurt. I'm clear headed.

It was astounding, quasi-mystical. I caught four more waves that day. After that, I was so disassembled. They took me home. They put me into bed. People had to bring me food for 14 days. The 15th was the day that I could move again. I got back in my car and I went back to the ocean and I did it again.

Over the course of about six months, when the only thing I was doing differently was surfing, I went from 10% functionality up to about 80%. I didn't know what the hell was going on. Worse, when I was surfing, I was having these quasi-mystical experiences in the waves. I'm a science guy. I don't have mystical experiences. Lyme disease, as you know, is only fatal if it gets into your brain.

I was certain that the Lyme had gotten into my brain. Even though I was feeling better, I thought I was losing my mind, and that I was actually dying. It started me on a giant quest to figure out what the hell was going on with me. Very quickly, I realized a couple of things about flow states.

One, they jack up the immune system. All the neurochemicals released in flow amplify the immune system. More importantly, to a guy with a chronic autoimmune condition like Lyme is this; your nervous system is going crazy. Flow resets the nervous system back to zero. It calms it back down. It's incredibly calm. All the normal stress chemicals in the brain, like cortisol and norepinephrine, get flushed out during a flow state. So the nervous system calms back down, which is why I came back to health.

Very quickly, I started to see the same things. Once I started to get these flow states while surfing, they started to show up when I was writing which was a big deal to me because I could work. I had bankrupted myself during that time to try to cure myself of Lyme. I couldn't work. There was no way to make money, but suddenly I got into these flow states while writing.

Flow is more like neuroplasticity if anything. You train it. The more flow you have, the more flow you have. The flow I was getting while surfing was helping me get into more flow while writing. Suddenly I went from half an hour a day of writing to four hours a day. I suddenly had a career again and I could begin to fight my way back.

This is a remarkable transformation. Steven Kotler has gone on to publish several New York Times bestselling books and continues to run the Flow Genome Project.

In my own experience with flow and its effect on my Meniere's disease symptoms, I have had several similar occurrences. When I first discovered Kotler's work, I had been suffering from constant brain fog, dizziness, and vertigo attacks for months. But I was finally starting to get a handle on my symptoms. I was also trying to come up with ideas for a product to invent and sell, to learn about product design, manufacturing, and online retail.

After deciding on the basic idea, I started trying to design a prototype. But after a couple of days, I hit a wall. I racked my brain but I couldn't figure out how to finish the design. Until one night, while getting ready for bed, my mind suddenly made a connection and I felt my brain kick into overdrive. I remember feeling a powerful sense of clarity. Colors suddenly seemed brighter. I was immediately flooded with ideas for my product, and by the time I went to bed, I had my design figured out entirely. I felt electric, invincible. I hadn't felt this good for months. My symptoms seemed to evaporate. When I woke up the next day, I no longer felt that lightning bolt of energy, but I didn't feel bad either. I felt much better than usual, and it lasted for several days. Creativity, it seemed, was my dominant flow trigger.

The Dark Side of Flow

I've had many experiences like this over the last couple years in varying degrees of intensity. When it does happen, it always feels so amazing. The feeling can be quite addictive. In *The Rise of Superman*, Kotler is quick to advise caution. He explains that all five of the neurochemicals that underpin the flow state are potent and addictive chemicals. Once you have experienced it, there is an incredible psychological draw that pulls a person towards flow. Additionally, flow occurs in cycles, and it is impossible to be in flow all the time. According to Kotler, "No question about it... there's a dark night of the flow. In Christian mystical traditions, once you've experienced the grace of God, the 'dark night of the soul' describes the incredible pain of its absence. The same is true for flow." I can personally attest to this. When the flow state eventually wears off, it can be incredibly frustrating. One day, you feel unstoppable. Everything is exciting, thoughts flow freely, and you can accomplish incredible things. Until suddenly it ends and you go back to normal. It can be an incredibly difficult transition, especially when your normal includes Meniere's disease.

What I can say is this: flow is the most powerful state of consciousness I have ever experienced and has shown me an aspect of human potential that I hadn't considered possible. As frustrating as it was to go from such a heightened state of being back to brain fog and dizziness, it filled me with hope. If a flow state was possible, and my symptoms disappeared in flow, then a return to health was also possible. In subtle ways, I have tried to shape my daily habits and environment around creating more flow in my life. It has been an amazingly positive force for healing and has helped me considerably to thrive.

Flow State Triggers

So if you want to experience flow and all the benefits it can provide, you're in luck. The Flow Genome Project has now identified 17 different flow state triggers and Steven Kotler has covered each one extensively in *The Rise of Superman*. Some are internally based while others are external and relate to your environment. He defines a flow trigger as a set of circumstances that enable you to quickly enter the flow state. I will briefly identify and introduce several of these triggers.

The first set of flow triggers are **psychological triggers**. There are four in total, and their purpose is to drive your awareness into the present moment, which is required for a flow state to occur.

The first psychological trigger is to maintain intensely focused attention. Very deep focus on one single, enjoyable task is often required to enter a flow state. The second psychological trigger is to have clear goals. When your goals are clearly defined, your mind knows exactly what it needs to do next, keeping you grounded in the present moment. The next psychological trigger is to have immediate feedback. If you are able to monitor your performance in real time, your brain doesn't need to analyze your past actions to decide what to do next. Instead, it can adapt and improve on the fly, again, keeping your focus on the present moment, on the task at hand. The final psychological flow trigger is to maintain the proper skill-to-challenge ratio. You want the task at hand to be challenging enough that you don't get bored, but not so challenging that you become frustrated.

The next set of triggers, known as **environmental flow triggers**, have to do with managing your external environment. The first trigger in this category is to have an environment with high consequences. When there is risk associated with a task, our brain often kicks into survival mode, which can quickly trigger a flow state. The next environmental flow trigger is to operate in a rich environment filled with novelty, complexity, and unpredictability. If you don't know what's coming next, you will pay much closer attention to your surroundings, keeping you in the present moment. The final environmental trigger is deep embodiment, or in other words, having a strong physical awareness of your environment. Maintaining an intimate awareness of, and connection to, your surroundings enables flow states to occur more frequently.

Creativity is a flow trigger and category all by itself. According to Kotler, when you look under the hood of creativity, you find pattern recognition and risk-taking. Both of these are elements of flow as well as flow triggers. Not to mention, creativity can produce flow, while flow, in turn, will greatly enhance your creativity.

The final set of flow triggers Kotler has identified have to do with altering our social lives and social environments to produce more flow as a group. These **social flow triggers** closely mirror the psychological flow triggers but are applied more broadly to increase flow in a group setting. If you have ever seen a major comeback at the end of a sports event, you have seen group flow in action. Group flow can also often be found in the workplace and is frequently associated with the startup culture. A 10-year study conducted by McKinsey & Company found that top executives are 500% more productive during flow. Though group flow is an important dynamic to consider, it is not directly relevant to your Meniere's disease treatment efforts.

To help you discover your dominant flow trigger, check out the Flow Genome Project's flow profile questionnaire at Flowgenomeproject.com. It only takes five minutes and will help you identify which triggers will most likely bring you into a flow state.

LIFESTYLE CHOICES

"You shouldn't focus on why you can't do something, which is what most people do. You should focus on why perhaps you can, and be one of the exceptions." – Steve Case

As you continue on your journey, there are many different lifestyle choices you can make to increase your quality of life and well-being. Once you have learned to live with your Meniere's disease, there are countless ways to grow and thrive as a happy and fulfilled member of society. To reach your potential as a person, it's important to always strive for improvement. Growth doesn't happen all at once. Usually, it's a slow and steady evolution of your character.

In his book *Man's Search for Meaning*, Holocaust survivor and psychologist Viktor Frankl writes, "I consider it a dangerous misconception of mental hygiene to assume that what man needs in the first place is equilibrium or, as it is called in biology, 'homeostasis,' i.e., a tensionless state. What man actually needs is not a tensionless state but rather the striving and struggling for a worthwhile goal, a freely chosen task. What he needs is not the discharge of tension at any cost but the call of a potential meaning waiting to be fulfilled by him." When we find ourselves simply coasting through life, there is little joy or excitement to be found. It's through concentrated effort that we can find happiness and a sense of purpose.

The rest of this chapter covers several important concepts to consider as you begin to design the new shape of your lifestyle.

Friends, Family, and Environment

Whether we like it or not, we are heavily influenced by the people closest to us. Our friends, family members, and coworkers all leave their mark on us in subtle ways. You may not realize it, but the people around you affect the decisions you make, the mannerisms in which you behave, and the mindset you adopt.

Understanding this offers the opportunity to design your environment for the best possible chance of success and happiness. But it also reveals the dark possibility that your inner circle of loved ones is doing you more harm than good. The legendary motivational speaker, Jim Rohn, used to say, "You are the average of the five people you spend the most time with."

Take a moment to reflect on this. Who are the five people closest to you? Are they positive, uplifting, and loving individuals who support you? Or are they negative and unpleasant, draining you of your life force, or constantly criticizing and putting you down?

Having Meniere's disease is hard enough. No one needs the added headache of a destructive support network. If your inner circle is less than ideal, I know how difficult it can be.

You don't get to choose your family and often it can feel like you're stuck. If a disruptive family member is unavoidable, the best advice I can offer is to establish clear boundaries and clear communication. Let them know you love them, but that you are struggling. Ask them to keep a positive tone and avoid criticism around you. Let them know that it will help you heal. It's strange, but sometimes people don't even realize the cycle of negativity they're caught up in until it's pointed out to them. If possible, minimize the time you spend with family members who bring you down.

Fortunately, we can choose our friendships. But, unfortunately, it can be incredibly difficult to cut ties with a long standing friend.

I look back at my life and wonder how I wasted so much time and energy on bad friendships. It's like I was a magnet for destructive people. I realize now that I was very much a people pleaser in my younger years, always trying to make everyone happy, but it was always at my own expense. It's a terrible trade-off to make.

Recently, I had to cut ties with an old friend. We got

along great for years, and he had really helped me through some difficult times in the past. But something had changed, and every time I was with him I would leave distraught. I was filled with stress and anxiety after spending any amount of time with him, and my symptoms started to get worse. The word "toxic" would flash across my consciousness.

When I finally cut ties, it didn't go well. In fact, it blew up in my face in a spectacular fashion. He didn't understand. First, he got defensive, but then he got angry, really angry. My response wasn't much better. I may be a reformed people pleaser, but I still hate confrontation. I pretty much shut down emotionally throughout the exchange. He stormed off in a rage.

But once the dust settled, the relief was palpable. I wish it could have played out differently, but I immediately felt so much better.

If a friendship or relationship is causing you distress, you need to get out. Like a bandage, rip it off fast. It hurts more initially, but the pain subsides much faster. You deserve to be happy, supported, and treated with respect. Make sure to choose your five people wisely. Be proud to be the average of those closest to you.

Passion, Momentum, and Motivation

Passion can be a powerful force for building momentum and motivation in your life, while

Meniere's disease and brain fog can quickly reduce both. The more momentum you have in reserve, the better. By discovering the things that you are passionate about, that get you fired up and excited to be alive, and pursuing them, you will be able to tap into a source of energy and love for life more powerful than anything you could have imagined.

So how do you find out what lights a fire under you? Well, it helps first to think back to your childhood. Before the world force-fed you an understanding of how life works. Before all your heartbreaks and pain. Before Meniere's disease. What did you love to do as a child? What did you want to be when you grew up? These questions will help get you thinking in the right direction.

Here is another good question to consider: If you never had to worry about money or illness, what would you do with your time?

Would you start a business? Create art? Make music? Help others, maybe work for a charity? Maybe you would write a book or a play or a memoir. Maybe you would learn a craft.

It's okay to not have the answers. Just asking the questions is a good start. My advice is simple: try lots and lots of new things. Expand your horizons as much possible, and when you find something that gets you excited, you may be on the right path. Even when your Meniere's symptoms limit you, there is still so much to explore and do on the internet from home, not to mention the days of relief from your symptoms. Take advantage of your good days to the fullest.

In my opinion, passion-fueled momentum is the most powerful force in the universe for counteracting brain fog. The raw, pure, unadulterated excitement that comes from working on a project that you are passionate about cannot be understated; treasure these moments. By following your passions, you are much more likely to enter flow states, as well.

As you explore new avenues of interest and begin to discover things that really fascinate you, I encourage you to dive deep. Follow that interest and see where it takes you. Make connections and find people who share your interest. Meetup.com is a fantastic resource to find like-minded individuals. Read books and watch documentaries. When you find that one thing that really sets your mind on fire, that gets you excited to wake up in the morning, you'll know you are on the right track.

By finding your passions and shaping your life around them to the best of your ability, you will not only reduce Meniere's ability to affect you, but you will discover a level of satisfaction and fulfillment that you may have never experienced before.

Cultivate a Love of Learning

Over the years with Meniere's disease, one of the things that helped me considerably was cultivating a love of learning. For so many of us, we have a tendency to go through our days like robots mindlessly following a script. We go to work, we come home, we watch TV, and we play on our iPhones, and browse Facebook. Distractions rule our lives.

I have found that engaging your mind with intellectual stimulation can do wonders to not only mitigate the effects of brain fog, but to expand your horizons considerably, as well. For me, this has taken a specific shape. I read as much as possible, often for several hours a day. I listen to interesting TED talks, interviews, and podcasts, and from time to time I take online courses to learn new skills.

I have found that by constantly feeding my mind interesting knowledge on topics that fascinate me, my mind seems to be sharper and less impacted by brain fog. When brain fog does occur, listening to an audio book or watching an interesting documentary is generally a good way to get my mind revved up and firing again.

It is also a great way to discover the new ideas that might spark your interest. It helps you to make new connections and find ways to improve your life, your work, and your hobbies. It will broaden your experiences and enable you to relate more deeply to more people.

Make time in your routine for intellectual stimulation. Learn that new skill you've always wanted to learn. Start reading that stack of books or novels that has been accumulating dust on your shelf. Fire up Netflix and watch an interesting documentary. Figure out what fascinates you, explore, and be inspired; it will build up your mental energy.

There is a world of possibilities larger than you can imagine, even if you are still struggling with your symptoms. Make it a goal to expand your mind as much as possible. You can accomplish anything you set your mind to.

CONCLUSION

"Most of the important things in the world have been accomplished by people who have kept on trying when there seemed to be no hope at all." – Dale Carnegie

My life has never really gone according to plan. Every time I thought I had it all figured out, my whole world would shift suddenly, dumping a new reality in my lap. But as challenging as my life has been at times, I wouldn't change a thing. This is a relatively new awareness for me, and when I look deep down inside myself, I know it's the truth. As I reminisce on my journey, the image of a pinball machine comes to mind; the small steel ball, violently bouncing off bumpers and walls, but invariably ending up in the right place.

A part of me still wonders what life would be like without Meniere's disease. A much larger part of me has high hopes that one day, science and medicine will answer that question. The largest part of me, however, realizes that ultimately life happens, and whatever happens, the best we can do is make the most of the hand we've been dealt.

Meniere's disease has given me an interesting perspective on life. I was diagnosed in my early twenties at a time when the invincible feeling of youth had yet to leave me. Meniere's disease delivered a lifetime dose of mortality directly into my brain. It was a hard pill to swallow, but I grew up quickly and faced the challenge head on. It's unfortunate that it took a terrible chronic illness to get me to accept responsibility for myself, but my accelerated maturity has paid off. Although I am not cured of Meniere's disease, I often feel blessed. I have a loving and supportive family, I'm getting married to an amazing woman, and I have found my calling in entrepreneurship.

From time to time, I still deal with my Meniere's symptoms, but I haven't had a vertigo episode in years. I feel healthier and happier now than I can remember being in a long time. No matter where you are in your treatment, no matter what setbacks or adversities you might face in your journey, you can start taking steps towards health. Even baby steps will get you there eventually. You can learn to live with this disease and find a sense of purpose, happiness, and clarity. You can prosper and thrive in your own way and create a life worth living to the fullest.

I wish you the best of luck in your journey, and above all else, remember: Meniere's disease will never define you. It cannot and will not ever be bigger than your dreams.

Resources

Mind over Meniere's Book Resources:
Mindovermenieres.com/Bookresources
An up-to-date listing of all the important links and resources found throughout this book.

The Mind over Meniere's Blog:
Mindovermenieres.com
The homepage of the Mind over Meniere's Blog. I post new articles weekly. Sign up for the Mind over Meniere's newsletters to stay up to date with all of my work.

The Mind over Meniere's Facebook Page:
Facebook.com/mindovermenieres
I post all of my new articles, as well as news from across the Meniere's disease community. Click "Like" to follow along.

The Mind over Meniere's Symptom Trigger Tool:
Mindovermenieres.com/Journal
A fillable, 1-page, PDF tool that I created to help you track your lifestyle and discover the unique triggers of your symptoms. It is completely free. Grab yours today!

The Vestibular Disorders Association (VEDA):

Vestibular.org

I have worked with the Vestibular Disorders Association for a while now as an Ambassador board member. They are an incredible nonprofit organization, and go above and beyond for the Meniere's disease community on a regular basis. For almost 30 years, VEDA has been a highly respected source of scientifically credible information on vestibular disorders. Through their publications and online community, VEDA has reached literally millions of vestibular patients with critical information and support.

I highly recommend getting involved, either by becoming a supporting member, or as a volunteer. You can help make a difference.

Meniere's Resources Inc.:

Menieresresources.org

Another great nonprofit organization that tirelessly serves the Meniere's disease community, day in, day out. Meniere's Resources Inc. is dedicated to raising public awareness about Meniere's disease and providing support and encouragement to those still suffering from Meniere's and other vestibular disorders.

The Ménière's Awareness Project:

Facebook.com/menieresawarenessproject

The Ménière's Awareness Project is a global support group, led by Judy McNamara Tripp, with a mission to shed light on those still suffering from Meniere's disease. I encourage you to click "Like" and follow along.

The Meniere's Disease Team:

Facebook.com/Menieresdisease

The Ménière's Disease Team is a global community dedicated to increasing awareness and advancing the development of new treatments for people living with Ménière's disease. They post news and helpful and inspirational content on a daily basis, as well as information on Meniere's disease clinical trials.

Facebook Support Groups

Meniere's Disease Support Group:
This is the Facebook-based support group that I run.
Facebook.com/groups/MenieresDiseaseSupportGroup

Meniere's Support Group:
Facebook.com/groups/4722666308

Meniere's: Stay Positive:
Facebook.com/groups/menieresstaypositive

Meniere's Disease Forums:

Meniere's Talk Forum:
Menieres.org

Daily Strength: Meniere's Disease Forum
Dailystrength.org/c/Menieres-Disease/forum

Looking to the Future:
New Research into Meniere's Disease

For the first time in a long time, there is real progress being made in Meniere's disease research, the development of new treatments, and new drug delivery systems.

Dr. López-Escámez: A Meniere's disease researcher out of Grenada, Spain, who is conducting ground breaking research into Meniere's disease. You can find an article I have written on Dr. López-Escámez's work here: Mindovermenieres.com/menieres-disease-one-mans-mission-to-find-a-cure

Otonomy (Otonomy.com): In 2008, Jay Lichter, Ph.D., a partner at Avalon Ventures and biotechnology industry veteran, experienced his first severe attack of vertigo. While driving, he became severely disoriented and had to pull to the side of the road. After multiple doctor visits, he was diagnosed with Ménière's disease and quickly experienced the limitations of available treatments. With his physician, Jeffrey Harris, M.D., Ph.D., chief of the division of otolaryngology-head and neck surgery at the University of California, San Diego, and several other experts in the field of otology, Dr.

Lichter founded Otonomy to bring new treatment options to patients with ear disorders.

Their mission today remains the same – to develop and commercialize novel and best-in-class therapeutics to address the significant unmet medical needs of patients with disorders of the ear.

Bibliography

Altucher, Claudia. *Becoming an Idea Machine: Because Ideas are the Currency of the 21st Century*. Choose Yourself Media, 2014.

Braun, Adam. *The Promise of a Pencil: How an Ordinary Person Can Create Extraordinary Change*. New York: Scribner, 2014.

Csikszentmihalyi, Mihaly. *Flow: The Psychology of Optimal Experience*. New York: HarperCollins, 1990.

Dweck, Carol. *Mindset: The New Psychology of Success.* New York: Random House, 2006.

Ferriss, Timothy. *The 4-Hour Work Week: Escape 9-5, Live Anywhere, and Join the New Rich*. New York: Crown Publishers, 2007.

Frankl, Viktor. *Man's Search for Meaning*. Boston: Beacon Press, 1959.

Holiday, Ryan. *The Obstacle is the Way: The Timeless Art of Turning Trials into Triumph*. New York: Penguin Group, 2014.

Kotler, Steven. *The Rise of Superman: Decoding the Science of Ultimate Human Experience.* New York: New Harvest, 2014.

Pollan, Michael. *The Omnivore's Dilemma: A Natural History of Four Meals.* New York: Penguin Group, 2006.

Stevenson, Shawn. *Sleep Smarter: 21 Proven Tips to Sleep Your Way to a Better Body, Better Health and Bigger Success.* Self-published, 2014.

ABOUT THE AUTHOR

Glenn Schweitzer is a small business owner, entrepreneur, and the creator of the popular Mind over Meniere's Blog. He is passionate about helping others with vestibular disorders and volunteers as an Ambassador Board Member for the Vestibular Disorders Association (VEDA). His articles have been read by tens of thousands of Meniere's disease sufferers in over 140 countries worldwide. He continues to raise awareness for Meniere's disease and spread his message of hope to those in need.